ONE MEAL A DAY INTERMITTENT FASTING

The Powerful Secret of the OMAD Diet for
Extreme Weight Loss

LOGAN WOLF

The only person you are destined to become is the person you decide to be.

Ralph Waldo Emerson

Table of Contents

____

Disclaimer

____

The purpose of writing this book is to educate the readers about the benefits of intermittent fasting. This book does not intend to give medical advice to any individual in any way. It should not be taken as a substitute for medical advice.

One Meal a Day (OMAD) routine of intermittent fasting requires a substantial lifestyle change. You must consult your physician before adopting any such measure for weight loss or any such benefit.

The author of this book is not a medical doctor or practitioner but has wide experience in intermittent fasting. The information given in the book is based on the personal experiences of the author and the information collected from other sources like the internet, books, and information videos.

The author or publisher of the book cannot be held liable for direct or indirect losses or damages of any kind due to the things mentioned in the book.

You must always take the advice of your doctor before incorporating any such change into your lifestyle. This book is not intended for medical advice.

The brands or trademarks if used in the book are only for clarification purposes and are owned by the owners themselves.

Images from pixabay.com

Congratulations on purchasing this book and thank you for doing so. This book will discuss the ways in which you can use One Meal a Day Intermittent Fasting for Extreme Weight Loss.

One Meal a Day (OMAD) may sound a bit intimidating. The idea of not having anything to eat for the whole day and eating all in one meal can be too much. If this thought also grips you, then you are not to be blamed. Our eating patterns have changed quite a bit in the last few centuries. We have food all around us, and this easy availability has led to incessant munching. Believe it or not, but it has caused more damage to our bodies than scarcity of food ever did. We are sitting on the ticking time bomb of obesity. It is not an impending disaster but a current one. It is an absurd yet scary fact that in spite of all the modern medical aid available today, more than 70% of the US population is overweight, and this isn't a pleasing number.

Obesity is a problem caused by various factors, but overconsumption of the wrong food at the wrong time is primary one among them. There are several ways to control this obesity epidemic, but overeating food cannot the answer. Intermittent fasting has emerged as a great solution to overcome obesity. One Meal a Day (OMAD) is an intermittent fasting practice that has gained quite a fame for its miraculous effects on weight.

'One Meal a Day' is one of the best ways to live a healthy life. It can help you in losing weight and in getting rid of several metabolic and lifestyle disorders. Obesity has spread its wings as an epidemic lately. As per the 2015-16 Center for Disease Control and Prevention (CDC) stats 39.6% of adults in the US are not just overweight, but obese. This is a scary number. Obesity limits the life choices of the victim to a great degree. It is a problem that can wreak havoc on the victim's personal, social, and professional life.

An obese person faces several metabolic issues and the options to an enjoyable life are drastically limited. There are physiological as well as psychological aspects of obesity that only the obese can understand.

The society can easily mock an obese person as someone who lacks the conviction to turn their life around. Low self-esteem is a rider that comes with obesity. Obese people are ripe cases for problems like hypertension, diabetes, osteoarthritis, cardiovascular diseases and other scary issues. They are constantly ridiculed for not having control over their eating urges. They are also on the receiving end of frequent advice to work out and lose weight. However, only a person suffering from obesity knows that these options don't really work out. While the advice sounds reasonable, it's not particularly helpful. Weight in itself is a debilitating factor. Working out with so much weight is not that easy as it is for fit people. Controlling their appetite becomes difficult and painful in their normal routine due to significant biological factors. The odds are never really in their favor.

Does this mean that they don't have options? No, it doesn't.

There are several examples where even extremely obese people have turned their lives around. It was challenging, but they did it. This means that it can be achieved. Can anyone do it? Hypothetically speaking, yes. Practically, no. Everyone can attempt to pump iron in the gym for 10 hours a day and build a body that people would die for. However, only a handful of people are can actually to do it.

It is also a myth that weight loss methods don't work. However, the same weight loss methods don't work for everyone. The only reason behind failures and successes is the amount of effort. This can't be the same for everyone. Therefore, you can't expect everyone to turn their lives around by traditional weight loss measures. Many of those methods aren't even practically viable for obese people in general. They do not answer even the primary indicator of success, long-term sustainability.

Who will benefit from this book?

This book is about a sustainable way to lose weight for obese people. This way will work even if your weight doesn't let you work out in the gym. It will work even if you have lost all hope of losing weight ever. You can lose much weight and lose it fast.

If you feel that your weight has limited your life choices and it is degrading you as a person, then this book is for you.

If you feel that now is the time to lose the weight and live a healthy life, then this book is especially for you.

If you feel that nothing has ever worked for you, then this book is just for you.

You will get to know the OMAD routine and the science behind it. This book will tell you the natural ways in which you can incorporate this routine into your life and get freedom from the life-limiting weight.

OMAD is the key to a healthy and happy life. You can lose weight fast and lose it safely.

You will not be taking any pills and won't need to pump iron in the gym for hours if you don't want to. This routine increases your metabolism and makes losing weight easy and fast.

No gain comes without some pain. You will have to put specific controls in place. However, they wouldn't be difficult, and with time they will become involuntary and natural. OMAD is a natural and time-tested way of intermittent fasting. It gives excellent results in quick weight loss. You will not only lose a substantial amount of weight but easily maintain it too.

If you have a hectic lifestyle and you don't get time to work out, OMAD will work for you. If you have reservations about leaving some kinds of foods entirely, OMAD will work for you. If you even have apprehensions about taking medications for weight loss, OMAD will work for you.

This book will be your detailed guide to OMAD Intermittent Fasting. It will walk you through the science behind OMAD and the things that make it so effective.

It will also clear the apprehensions about your ability to follow it. It will tell you the specific advantages of OMAD.

You will also get to know the detailed process of adopting the OMAD routine in your life.

This is a comprehensive guide to the One Meal a Day intermittent fasting, and I am sure it will change your perspective about losing weight altogether.

One Meal a Day (OMAD) is the most sustainable and remarkable way for you to lose weight, even if all other measures have failed. However, you will have to put yourself together. In obese people, losing the weight is not the only challenge, maintaining it is an even bigger problem. People who go under the knife for weight reduction surgeries find themselves standing in the same place soon. One Meal a Day will not only help you in losing a lot of weight fast, but it will also assist you in maintaining it effortlessly.

You need to read the book carefully and understand the effects of intermittent fasting on your body. The mechanics of food plays a critical role in our bodies and the One Meal a Day routine brings harmony to it. This book will help you in establishing a symbiotic relationship between your food and your body.

There are plenty of books on this subject on the market, so thank you again for choosing this one! Every effort was made to ensure it is full of as much useful information as possible. Please enjoy!

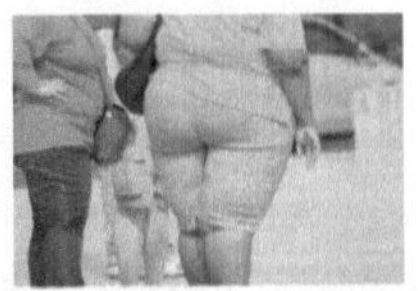

The Reasons for Current Obesity Epidemic

OBESITY HAS TAKEN the form of an epidemic in modern society. The facts are a clear indicator that we are not learning or improving at all. In the year 1962, on average 13.4% of people were found to be obese in the US. The percentage of people suffering from extreme obesity was very low standing at 0.9%. However, over the years, the increase in this percentage is staggering. In the year, 2016, 39.6% of people suffered from Obesity, and out of these over 9% were extremely obese.

More than 70% of adults in the US are either overweight or obese. It means that more than 2 out of three US adults suffer from weight issues. This doesn't paint a very pretty picture. The escalating rate of increase in obesity is another cause of concern. In 1997, only 39.4% of people were overweight in the US. This saw a rise of 5% in 2004, and again increased by 12% in the next three years until 2007. A decade later the total percentage of overweight people in the US has gone past 70%.

The rate of obesity in women is even scarier. Data shows that the rate of obesity among women has risen steeply in the past four decades in comparison to men.

The number of preventable deaths in the US is 900,000 every year. Out of these, more than 400,000 people die due to obesity-related disorders. Restraining this menace of obesity would have prevented most of these losses .

However we may brood about the situation of obesity in the country, the fact stands that third parties have no significant role to play in it. Our wrong choices have led to this epidemic of obesity. The only way out is to improve those choices. Aggressive marketing by food companies, fast-paced lifestyles, stress, and anxiety may take the blame, but still, the bulk of the problem has been on our end.

When it is the time to take responsibility, we try to find an easy target. Food is the easy scapegoat. It is the natural suspect. People easily blame food and eating habits of the victim to obesity. Although it cannot be denied that food is among the chief reasons for causing obesity, however, it is not the lone wolf.

There can be reasons for obesity in which victims do not have much control. Hormonal imbalance, genetic issues, and other such medical problems can lead to abnormal and uncontrolled weight gain. However, many times, it is just our carelessness that leads to excessive weight gain.

MAJOR FACTORS other than food that lead to obesity

Stressful Life

The stressful life of the modern world is a significant contributor to weight gain. Stress leads to an urge to relax. Certain kinds of products like artificial sweeteners, processed foods, chocolates, alcohol, and nicotine, are used in an effort to reduce stress and relax. However, most of these items, as well as stress, are bad for health. We may blame the obesity on these items, but ultimately, stress it what leads to these indulgences. You become lethargic and stop venturing out. You shirk all physical activities. The extra calories in these products start piling up. Your brain gets slow, and you accumulate weight.

Lack of Time

The hectic life is another reason for dangerous weight accumulation. We are running so fast and so mindlessly that we have lost focus. The need for speed stops us from focusing on even the basic requirements of life, (i.e. healthy food). We start jumping on fast foods to save time. It is cheap and fast—both things nature never wanted food to be. When you start getting such a vital thing so quickly, and effortlessly, you stop thinking about it. Fast foods are full of empty calories and lack most critical nutrients. They are fattening, carcinogenic, inflammatory and lead to craving. This mindless eating leads to excessive weight gain.

Lack of Physical Activity

Lack of physical activity is another big problem. Earlier, we had to fight and put our lives at stake to earn food, but that's a thing of fables now. Money can buy food today, and you need to sweat separately to burn that food. This isn't easy for many. Some don't have that kind of time and luxury; others lack the motivation for it. The little time that's left with them is again spent on eating.

WE SEE that most of these factors are a result of something else. The food is at the bottom of it, but it is not the only reason weight gain begins.

However, it is also a notable fact that there has been a shift towards the kind of food items we eat these days. The healthy unprocessed food items have been replaced by ready to eat foods. They taste great but are mostly garbage for your body. They fill you with empty calories, lead to weight gain and cause inflammation. We are well aware of them, yet we choose to ignore them.

A big reason for such attraction towards wrong food items is the excessive marketing by the food producing companies. These companies are earning billions by selling you such food products. You feel good by eating them, and therefore you believe everything they say without thinking twice. This leads to the obesity epidemic. They are hammering you night and day with a single motive. They want you to buy their product. They are simply telling you that you can lose weight by eating their products.

Take a deep breath here. Does this not sound ridiculous? You can lose weight by eating things. Really?

Let's do simple math. Food means calories. There is nothing that doesn't add weight except water. The low-calorie foods fill you with artificial sweeteners, harmful fats, and other more dangerous things. They cause weight gain and a lot of it. The label only serves to mislead you.

Therefore, when you eat anything, you are adding calories. However, you are not doing anything out of the ordinary to burn those calories. There is no way that your weight will go down by eating them. On the contrary, those extra calories, fat, and sweeteners will cause more damage.

If someone expects that weight loss will occur without any sacrifice, then he or she are in a delusion and need to wake up.

If someone thinks that starting a rigorous diet routine will lead to weight loss, then 9 out of 10 times, the end is sad, as people are not able to retain the rigorous diets for long. The day they start eating their normal diet, they begin binge eating. They try to compensate for the loss of all the time they couldn't eat on their wish.

If someone expects that he or she'll get "fat to fit" by pumping iron in the gym for a month and flaunt the Adonis-like body, then he or she should stop living in a fairytale. It's not going to work out. First, it is not easy for most, especially for obese people for obvious reasons. Second, the day they get back to their regular routine, the gym starts looking tough. The lost weight comes back much faster.

The weight loss industry is thriving on this. In the U.S. alone, the weight loss industry generated a profit of $66 billion in 2017, yet the percentage of people suffering from obesity has increased this year.

The reason is plain and simple. It isn't working sustainably. There is no problem with the weight loss measures. You can temporarily lose weight through every method. You either go on a diet, do yoga, dance, exercise, or pump iron in the gym. You will burn calories. When the number of calories burnt in a day exceeds the amount of calories consumed in that day, you will lose some weight.

The real problem is with sustainability. You are not able to carry on most of these activities for long. As soon as you get back to your usual routine, the weight starts piling on.

Intermittent fasting and especially the OMAD technique are here to help you with this specific problem. It is the sustainable way to lose weight. You are not required to do things out of the ordinary. You can and will follow your regular schedule. You do not need to cut out your working hours for hitting the gym. You do not need to restrict your diet extensively. You can eat pretty much anything as long as it is healthy. You merely need to regulate the timing of when you eat.

The timing is of the essence in intermittent fasting. It gives your body the chance to focus on the fat stores in your body. It also ensures that you do not pile up your body with extra calories as you get a very short window to eat. Although you can eat pretty much anything in that window, biology takes over in that period. Your appetite comes into control, and your eating pattern is regulated.

The next few chapters will explain in detail the behavior of your hunger hormones and satiety. You'll learn that the craving you always had for food is not because of the urge to eat but due to the imbalance in your body that can be corrected. You will also learn that regulating your food intake is an easy and straightforward task. You'll even get to know the impact of insulin on your body and the wonders that controlling your blood sugar can do.

Intermittent fasting is not just a weight control measure but a way of life. You can get the benefits of a healthy life and body by making some simple changes to the way you eat and you can lose much weight very quickly. The OMAD routine is the key to quick weight loss, and it is a natural and sustainable measure.

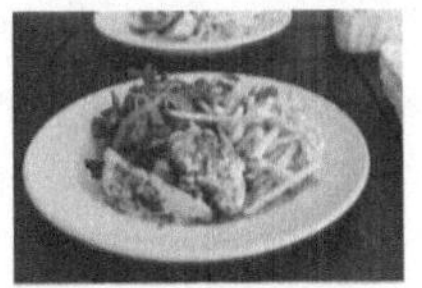

2

What is One Meal a Day?

FOR THE SAKE OF SIMPLICITY, One Meal a Day (OMAD) is the same as it sounds. You can have one complete meal in a day and will have to fast for the next 23 hours in this intermittent fasting routine. Before we move further on this concept, it is also important to understand 'Intermittent Fasting'.

Intermittent fasting is a pattern of eating. It means that you have specified 'Fasting' and 'Eating' windows and you have to follow a disciplined routine. The numbers of hours you fast will vary upon the kind of 'routine' you choose. 'Routine' is a crucial word here. The absence of a routine is the reason behind the failure of most weight-loss measures. Therefore, practicing intermittent fasting as a routine or a lifestyle is very important for good results.

One Meal a Day (OMAD) is among the several routines you can follow in intermittent fasting. However, it is one of the best methods for fast and extreme weight loss.

The basic requirement of OMAD is that you will have to fast for 23 hours and then you can have one big meal, preferably in the evening. The evenings are great for one big meal as your day has a fulfilling end. In this meal, you will be free to eat practically anything that you like. However, it is always prudent to choose healthy and balanced food as you are going to draw all your nutrition from this meal. This is one of the most favored methods of extreme weight loss and lean muscle gain even for body-builders. It helps in shedding body fat and gaining lean muscle mass.

You can have only one full meal in the day. Therefore, the food should have the right mix of carbohydrates, fat, protein, and fiber. Nevertheless, you can include items for which you have a craving. For instance, eating sweets, cakes and cookies are okay with this routine as long as you follow the 23-hour food curfew.

Some people might start getting anxious right away at the thought of not being able to eat for 23 hours. The fear of starvation and hunger pangs will have started kicking in. Although their concerns may seem logical, they are unwarranted. You can choose the speed with which you implement intermittent fasting. The transition to the OMAD routine should be slow and well adapted. We will discuss this in detail in later chapters.

OMAD is no doubt a strict routine to endure. However, it will yield great results. OMAD routine will help you in burning the fat stores more efficiently and quickly.

The transition to OMAD is not very tough, as you do not need to begin with the 23 hours fasts from the very first day. You will start with smaller fasts as 16:8 and then move ahead to 20:4 and finally to 23:1. This means, in the beginning, you can fast for 16 hours and then eat 2-3 meals in the remaining 8 hours. Once you get used to it and become comfortable with this routine, you can move ahead with the 20 hours fast and 4 hours of eating window. The last step in this process is the 23 hours fast and 1-hour eating window. To an outsider, it may look like a very restrictive regimen, but in reality, it isn't.

People are usually very concerned about the hunger pangs while fasting. However, your hunger pangs are not a result of your need for food but are caused by several other factors like the habit of eating and inflammation in the fat cells. Once you start practicing intermittent fasting, these issues are taken care of by your body itself. You'll notice that your need for food is not as controlling as you always believed.

Intermittent fasting and especially the **OMAD** routine bring many benefits along with it, and the best one is extreme weight loss.

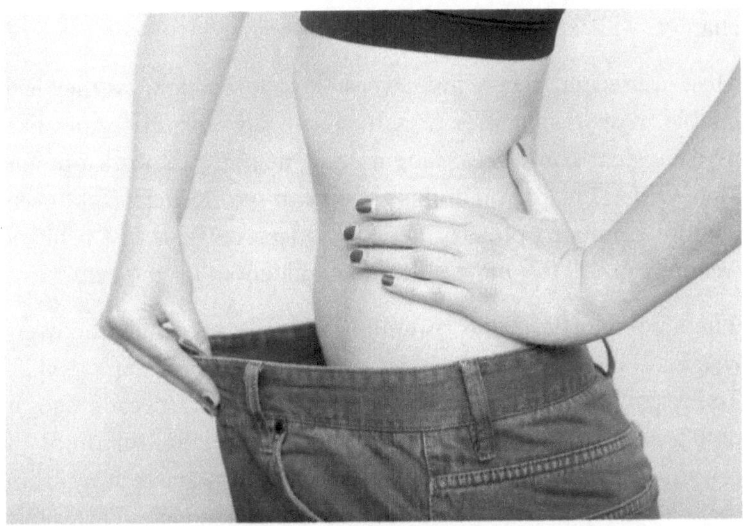

Firstly, intermittent fasting is one of the safest and most reliable ways to lose weight.

Secondly, you can lose weight by the **OMAD** routine even if your weight issues restrict you from working out initially.

Thirdly, you will not have to abandon the foods you love. This is among the primary reasons other diet programs fail, as people are not able to resist the foods they love for very long.

Fourthly, it is easy to make this routine a part of your lifestyle. This gives the routine sustainability. You will lose weight and keep it off too. Weight regain is a big issue with people who lose a considerable amount of weight quickly. This won't happen with OMAD. There won't be a weight relapse.

OMAD routine will help you in losing weight and staying in shape. It will help you in losing weight even if you are unable to work out initially due to excessive weight. However, workouts will help once you lose weight and will help you not only in losing weight more quickly but also with skin tightening. The later chapters will explain the science behind this.

Most overweight people are never able to lose weight, as they feel unable to work out in the gym. There are several factors like psychological complexes, fatigue, and inability to work out for long. OMAD helps you in this as you can start losing weight even without strenuous physical activity. Once you have lost a bit of weight, you will feel more able and confident to hit the gym.

The anxiety of fasting is common in people, especially the overweight. They feel that staying away from food is impossible. Today's youth feels the same for social media. A decade ago, it didn't even exist, and humanity had survived for hundreds of centuries without it. Just one generation ago, staying away from the TV was impossible, yet humankind had survived. This is just like the fear of cold you experience before entering the water. Once inside, you don't want to get out of it. Centuries ago, our ancestors lived on only 'One Meal a Day' as the food was scarce, yet they thrived. Food has become our habit; it isn't a necessity of our body in the quantities we consume it.

The daily calorie needs of any healthy individual can be consumed easily even in one meal. We are overloading our system by taking several meals a day, and we can see by the obesity stats that it isn't helping.

As far as the hunger pangs are concerned, in most cases, they either are a result of your habit of eating or are caused by inflammation in the fat cells. Regular eating creates an imbalance in our hunger and satiety hormones, and this leads to frequent cravings for food. Once you start intermittent fasting, things come into harmony, and your body regulates these hormones. Your hunger pangs will subside quickly. There are several measures to suppress these hunger pangs without consuming calories that will help you initially. We'll discuss all these measures in detail in the coming chapters. We will also examine how the hunger and satiety hormones function and ways to balance them.

The OMAD routine is straightforward. It has no complexities involved. You get to choose the time you want to eat. It can be morning, evening or afternoon. The choice is up to you. The only rule of the routine is that you can have only one full meal and that's it. It will be your body that will be working overtime to burn the excess fat in your body. The how and why of the process are explained in detail in the upcoming chapters.

Therefore, if you are troubled by your excess weight then read the coming chapters very carefully.

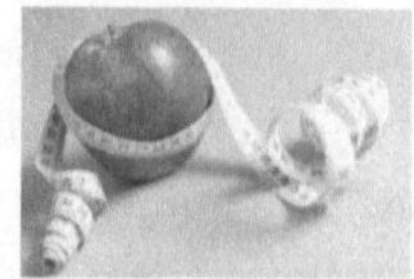

3

How the OMAD Routine Works

WEIGHT LOSS IS A COMPLEX PROCESS. As the saying goes, "Rome wasn't built in a day," and the same goes for your accumulated weight and fat. The excess weight and fat have been piling on for a long time. Mostly, fat accumulation is a result of your negligence about your lifestyle choices. Here, considering the word 'mostly' is key, as it is not the sole reason that can lead to weight gain.

Genetic problems, other health issues leading to immobility and hormonal issues can also lead to weight gain. However, this book is about the weight gain issues in individuals who have gained excess weight and belly fat due to poor lifestyle choices. Therefore, we'll stick to it.

Our body has a very sophisticated and detailed system of functioning. It is crucial that you comprehend the way our body functions to understand the causes that lead to excess weight gain. The first concept to grasp is that your body doesn't consider the weight as a liability but an asset.

Like all other organisms on this blue planet, human beings were also created to survive for long periods. The food is a prized commodity for all creatures, and so it was for humankind. In the beginning and, until the past few centuries, getting food was not that easy. Men had to put up a fight against beasts to get every morsel of food. It was tough, and there was no certainty. There were seasons of feasts and famines. Our body has a system of accumulating energy in the form of fat to survive the times of famines. This fat is used in times when there is no supply of food. This mechanism is still used for all other beings. However, there has been a slight change for humankind in this regard. The seasons of famines have almost ceased to exist thanks to the abundance of food brought by modernization. This mechanism is still in place and functioning.

When you eat anything, your body processes that food into the form of glucose. Your body then assesses the current need for energy. The required energy passes into your bloodstream in the form of blood glucose. All your organs and cells can access this as direct energy. Your pancreas gets to work and releases the hormone insulin that helps the cells to absorb this energy. However, when the produced energy is more than is required our body stores that extra energy in the form of glycogen. This is directly stored in the liver and muscles. The insulin present in your blood will direct this transformation. However, when the present energy is much higher than the amount which can be stored in the form of glycogen, it needs to be stored as fat. Insulin sends signals to the fat stores and places the extra energy in the form of fat cells. This is the process of accumulation of visceral fat, the fat around your belly, thighs, hips, and all the odd places.

Now, there is a fundamental question here. When our body has such an efficient system, why doesn't it target this fat on its own? Why is burning this visceral fat so tricky? Here, you will have to return to the earlier point that our body is following the feast and famine system. The fat stores in the body are not a liability, but an asset for our body. Our body tries to keep the fat stores intact to be used in the rainy days when food is scarce. However, those days rarely come in modern society. In today's reality, that fat is a liability to you. Your body will never try to burn these fat stores on its own until it necessarily feels the need to do so.

The fact is clear that your body will not burn this body fat until it is forced to do so. If you believe that by dieting or exercising in the usual way you can force your body to burn this beloved fat, then you are mistaken. Your body will only take these steps when it feels that it is in short supply.

Our body will burn the tough visceral fat only when it is in dire need of energy. This can't happen while you keep feeding it with more and more food at regular intervals. Therefore, intermittent fasting is the best way to cut this continuous supply of readily available energy to our body. It helps you in forcing your body to start burning the fat stores that can supply clean energy to our body. However, there is a big misconception that intermittent fasting, or for that matter, any fasting can make you weak.

Once again, think of our ancestors. They were hunter-gatherer nomads. There was no surety of food for them. With their primitive weapons and limited knowledge, the odds of getting food on a daily basis were low. However, their bodies needed more strength on the days when they didn't have food for long periods, to hunt more aggressively. Their minds needed to think more clearly on the days they didn't get food. If not, their odds of getting any more food would reduce drastically. Therefore, the misconception that the lack of food for some time of fasting will make you weak or take away the clarity of thoughts is wrong. Once your ready supply of energy is cut-off, your body will switch to burning the fat for energy. It needs to be even stronger and more robust on those days to survive in a hostile environment.

Intermittent fasting is the way our bodies have been designed to function by Mother Nature. Your work schedule and type of job won't be a problem. Your energy needs are also no factor when considering intermittent fasting as you get the required amount of energy in your eating windows. The OMAD routine of intermittent fasting gives you an eating window so that you can get the supply of energy needed. This will ensure that your body doesn't feel it is in a starvation situation. Nevertheless, it will keep your body in a fasted state for long enough so that it feels the need to start burning the fat stores. Whether you are doing a white-collar job with a 9 to 5 shift or pumping iron in the gym for bodybuilding, intermittent fasting can work for all.

It is the best and most successful way to reduce weight and burn the tough belly fat. The OMAD routine gives your body a fasting window of 20+ hours. This fasting window helps in speeding up the weight loss and fat burning procedure.

The OMAD routine also has several other health benefits. It has incredible anti-aging benefits and improves your overall health biomarkers. This routine improves your insulin sensitivity and cures the chronic inflammation in the fat cells.

SOME FANTASTIC BENEFITS of the OMAD routine

- Improved Insulin Sensitivity
- Better Ghrelin Release
- Effective Leptin Sensitivity
- Immense HGH Boost
- Accelerated Metabolism
- Autophagy (cellular repair) is activated

- Relief from Chronic Inflammation in the Fat Cells
- Reduction in Cardiovascular Issues
- Reduction in Oxidative Stress and Free Radical Damage

The best thing about the OMAD routine is that it is sustainable. This term has been mentioned several times. The real significance of this term is that you can actually follow it for a long-term. This outcome is quite tricky to achieve in other weight loss methods.

People who don't have any experience of fasting of any kind feel quite intimidated by it. They think that fasting for so long would be next to impossible considering their current state. Some believe that the idea of staying hungry for so long would crush them, but believe me—you will have several things to worry about while on intermittent fasting. Your worries could range from old clothes not fitting you anymore, the added expense of buying new clothes, but hunger pangs wouldn't be one of the troubling issues.

Intermittent fasting and the OMAD routine is no magic trick. You will not be taking any special medicines or supplements. You will be rubbing no lotion on your tummy. All you would be doing is training your body to burn the excess fat for access to easy energy. This is one of the healthiest ways to lose weight. It's the reason your body has been storing fat all these years, to BURN it eventually.

To understand the process of losing weight through intermittent fasting and the OMAD routine, you will need to understand in detail the way our bodies function. The next few chapters will walk you through the whole process and tell you how you will benefit.

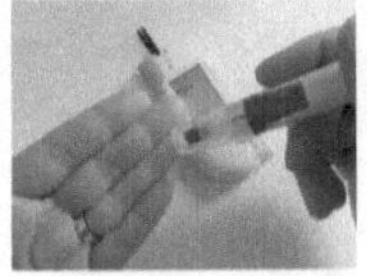

4

How it Improves Insulin Sensitivity

IF THERE IS one hormone that affects your weight the most, it is the insulin hormone. Our pancreas releases the insulin hormone as soon as the digested food comes into your bloodstream in the form of glucose. The insulin hormone functions as a key to your cells. Your cells cannot absorb glucose energy until insulin is present. This hormone enables the cells to absorb this blood glucose as a direct energy source.

Any food that you eat takes around 5-8 hours to process completely. This means that if you are living a so-called normal lifestyle, then you can consume 5-6 meals a day. Your day will start by eating breakfast in the morning, some snacks before noon, lunch in the afternoon, and snacks in the evening and dinner at night. In that case, you will always have a high blood glucose level. Your pancreas will always be at work and continuously producing insulin. This is a clear invitation to a dangerous condition called pre-diabetes.

If you do the math, limiting your calories is a tough task with so many meals to eat, even if you are eating carefully.

If your taste buds easily control you, then staying away from fast food will also be very difficult. This means that you will not only be eating more calories, but you'll also be consuming empty calories, added sugar, and unhealthy food.

Five to six meals a day means that your insulin levels would always remain spiked from absorbing so much energy from all the meals.

The insulin, although a vital hormone, can wreak havoc on your health when unregulated. Your pancreas can come under high stress when it has to work continuously for so long without a break. This is a hazardous situation.

Insulin is the most powerful fat storage hormone. This means that it tells your fat cells to store more and prevents them from breaking apart. Let us understand this procedure clearly.

Whenever you eat, your blood sugar levels increase as the energy derived from carbohydrates comes in the form of glucose. Your pancreas is the first to respond, and it releases insulin from the beta cells. The insulin binds to the cells and helps them in absorbing the required glucose. The extra energy is stored in the muscles and liver in the form of glycogen. However, when there is still excess, that energy is stored in the fat cells with the help of insulin. It is the primary hormone that is communicating with your fat cells and instructing them to store more fat.

When there is a steady supply of energy in the bloodstream, and insulin levels are always elevated, your body will never start burning fat cells. The insulin will always send a message that there is an abundant supply of energy and there is no need to burn fat.

In this state, if you exercise more, you will feel weak and drained as your body would keep sucking the readily available glucose in the blood but not affect your fat stores. If you follow a low-calorie diet, then also there would be a minimal effect, as the blood glucose levels would remain high. Your fat cells would never get the message, as there will be the barrier of insulin in between.

This is where the current mechanism fails. It doesn't matter how little or how healthy you are eating. If you were frequently eating, then your blood glucose supply would always be abundant. This means that the pancreas would have to keep pumping more and more insulin into your blood. This is the point where another problem starts which is called insulin resistance.

You must have heard 'familiarity breeds contempt.' This is true to a great extent as far as overexposure to insulin is concerned. When your blood sugar levels remain unusually high, your pancreas needs to keep pumping insulin at a faster pace. This causes inflammation in the cells, and they start responding to insulin with intensity, which means that although your pancreas is producing insulin, your cells react slowly to them when required. This means your pancreas will have to provide more insulin. It creates a vicious cycle.

THIS PROCESS IS SO bad that it can flush all your weight loss efforts down the drain. People with insulin resistance can have 5-7 times more insulin in their blood as compared to insulin sensitive people. The sad part is that this is not the end of it. Besides diabetes, there are other issues associated with high insulin levels in your blood. You cannot lose weight if your insulin levels are high, as it will keep sending the signals of surplus energy to your brain. It will also lead to stress.

When the insulin levels remain elevated for long, our body starts the chronic stress response. It sends a message of attack on your body and slows down the metabolism. The stress hormones give a push to the defensive mechanism. Your heart rate, cardiac output, and blood pressure will go up. Immunity, growth, repair, and similar mechanisms will take a back seat, and the body will start pumping out lots of cholesterol. The cholesterol is vital for the production of hormones in your body. This means that you will have not only high insulin levels but also high cholesterol levels. If you already have diabetes, then the problems have no end for you, and if don't, then it is at your doorstep. This is a big reason that obese people are at such a high risk of diabetes and other lifestyle disorders.

Regulating your insulin production is one of the most important steps towards effective weight management. Insulin is a hormone that not only prevents fat burning but also prohibits the production of other hormones that lead to weight loss and fat burning. One such important hormone is Human Growth Hormone (HGH).

HGH is an essential hormone as far as cutting your belly fat, and building muscle. If you are trying to trim your belly fat and build muscles, then this is the hormone for you. It can accelerate the whole process with unimaginable speed. It is a vital hormone responsible for most of your growth-related activities. However, production of this hormone is not possible as long as insulin is present in your blood. Insulin will remain present in your blood for 5-8 hours after your last meal. If you are taking short meals throughout the day, then it means that there can be no production of HGH at all.

Intermittent fasting and especially the OMAD routine ensure that you only have an eating window of 4 hours. You remain in a fasted state for around 20 hours. When you minus the 8 hours of insulin present in your blood, there are still 12 hours when your body is free to burn fat. After a few hours after your last meal, your body will start feeling the need for blood glucose to continue its operations. As you wouldn't have eaten anything for a long time, there would be no blood glucose. The body would look for alternative sources of energy, the glycogen stored in the liver and muscles. However, the glycogen stored in the muscles can't be utilized for the whole body as it is specifically for utilization by the muscles and the organs. The specific enzymes to make use of it are not present in general. This paves the way for burning the visceral fat, as it is the next significant source of energy. This is the time for which the body had been conserving energy.

Apart from the first couple of days when you start intermittent fasting, you won't feel weak or have other signs of fatigue. The reason is straightforward; the energy produced by the fat cells is potent and clean. It is capable of running your body smoothly. The first couple of days are the adjustment days. Your body is transitioning from burning energy produced by carbohydrates in your food to burning fat in the cells. Fat is a clean fuel for the body. It leaves no toxic waste, and you will not only feel more energetic and healthy but more relieved too.

Accumulation of fat cells around your vital organs causes several types of inflammation. You may not be able to feel it, but your organs always remain under stress. The continuous production of stress hormones makes you deficient in many things as your body is always on the defensive.

Once you start losing the abdominal fat, you will feel more energetic, lively, and fresh. The stress levels will go down, and you will be able to cope with diseases and situations even better.

The insulin resistance is a problem you would most certainly like to avoid. However, recent reports suggest that almost 50% of Americans are insulin resistant. A study published online in JAMA stated that more than 50% of the adults in the US are either suffering from diabetes or pre-diabetes. Obese people are at the highest risk of developing pre-diabetes as suggested in the same report. This all indicates that insulin resistance is becoming a big problem. It is an open invitation to a number of issues in your body, and it is a definite 'No Trespassing' sign for all fat burning efforts. You can help yourself by adopting intermittent fasting, as it is an easy and viable solution.

You can easily recover from insulin resistance and develop insulin sensitivity. Your body starts responding better to insulin in this state. This means your pancreas does not need to pump out more and more insulin. Your pancreas gets time to recover, and the insulin and blood glucose levels remain in control. You will be able to burn your fat faster and with greater ease.

This chapter explained to you how insulin affects our body and fat burning. It puts your body in a defensive mode. However, the provocative question of hunger is still looming large in the air. You may now have a healthy fear of too much insulin, but fear of staying hungry is still there. It is important to address this concern, as intermittent fasting cannot be done without being in a fasted state for extended periods.

The next chapter will shed light on your hunger mechanism and how it affects intermittent fasting.

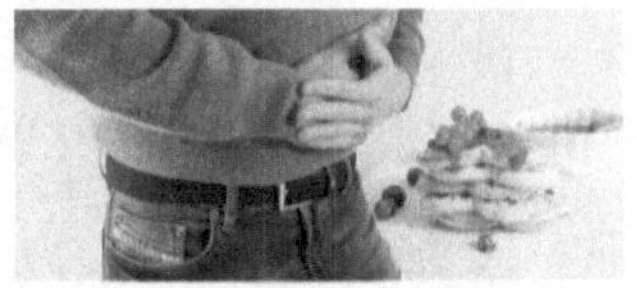

5

How it Normalizes the Hunger Hormone, Ghrelin

GHRELIN IS THE HUNGER HORMONE. When your stomach is empty, it releases the ghrelin hormone in large quantities. This hormone then sends signals to the hypothalamus of your brain to eat. In a healthy body, the ghrelin levels are at the peak when you have an empty stomach, and the levels start to drop as you eat. Around an hour after you have eaten the meal, the ghrelin release completely stops. You will not have any craving to eat anymore.

However, this is not the case with obese people. Their ghrelin release is never very high, nor very low. Before taking a meal, the ghrelin release in obese people is comparatively lower than it is for healthy people. Even after eating the meal, their stomach keeps releasing the ghrelin hormone is small quantities. This creates the whole problem of craving. You are never completely satisfied. You want to eat all the time. This frequent eating leads to excess weight gain.

Ghrelin is a crucial hormone. It not only regulates your hunger but also helps in the production of HGH. Frequent eating messes with the ghrelin release function. The low but constant release of ghrelin hormone confuses your brain about your hunger.

Intermittent fasting puts a stop to this confusion. You get a long fasting period in which your stomach is completely empty. Your stomach is then able to produce an ample amount of the ghrelin hormone. This hormone also helps in the production of HGH. If you work out in the fasted state, your body will be able to burn fat faster as there will be much HGH in your system.

Several studies have also found that the ghrelin hormone has a good impact on your memory and learning as well. You might have noticed that you can think better and work fast when you haven't eaten for some time. As soon as you eat, you start feeling lethargic and fuzzy.

Intermittent fasting is one of the best ways to normalize your ghrelin levels. It gives your body the time to develop hunger completely, and once you have taken a meal after a break, you will stop feeling hungry completely.

One important point to add here is that the kind of food you eat also has a powerful impact on your ghrelin release. If you eat healthy food with lots of fiber and nutrients, your ghrelin levels will be better. If you have a habit of eating a lot of processed food, fast food, and added sugars, then your ghrelin release will always be erratic.

Shakespeare once said 'a rose by any other name would smell as sweet.' I'm afraid that can't be said about the food items we eat. Fruits and vegetables that we eat contain glucose. Our body can quickly use this glucose in the form of energy. However, the added sugar that we eat contains fructose. It is also sugar like glucose, but our body cannot use it in the same manner. Only our liver can metabolize fructose and stores it as visceral fat. The process of metabolizing this glucose leads to the creation of a ton of toxic waste. The buildup of uric acid, high blood pressure, and gout are some of the harmful results of fructose consumption.

When you eat glucose, not even a fraction of it will be converted to fat, whereas a major portion of fructose is converted to fat.

Glucose consumption will directly lead to a lowering of the ghrelin level. However, your ghrelin levels would increase after the consumption of fructose.

Have you ever noticed that you still have a craving for food and drinks after you have had fast food and carbonated beverages? This is due to the presence of high amount of fructose in these items. Fructose is present in all kinds of processed foods with added sugar.

Some fruits also contain fructose but consuming them isn't unhealthy. They are rich in fiber and have lots of water. Chewing them negates most of the negative impact caused by fructose. On the other hand, eating processed food or carbonated beverages will cause considerable damage.

If you are aiming to lose weight, then wisely choosing your food items will be important. The food that creates cravings will make it difficult for you to remain in a fasted state.

You cannot lose weight by merely counting calories; you will also have to watch the kind of calories you are consuming. Eating a low carb diet will not only suppress your hunger and make you feel more satisfied it would also help your body to work correctly.

Intermittent fasting is for those people who have been in the habit of consuming too many empty calories. It will help you in normalizing your ghrelin levels and adjust them as per your routine. Higher levels of ghrelin in the fasted state will give you better clarity of thought and increase the production of HGH. It will also help in establishing harmony with your satiety hormone.

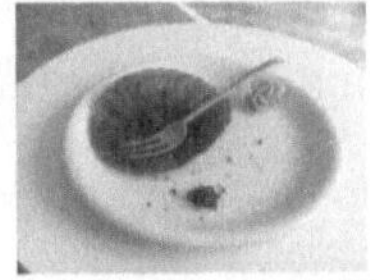

6

How it Improves Your Sensitivity to Leptin, Your Satiety Hormone

HORMONES from all parts of your body are sending signals to your brain all the time. These signals direct your brain to do the right things. Similarly, hormones are released by your fat cells too. The fat cells send messages to your brain that your fat storage is complete and you need to stop eating. This is a natural process, and those hormones are called Leptin.

The leptin hormone is also called the satiety hormone, and that's for a reason. Whenever you eat something, your body starts releasing leptin. An increase in leptin levels sends a signal to the hypothalamus of your brain that you have eaten enough and you should stop eating. Leptin and ghrelin levels should be inversely proportional. This means when you are hungry your ghrelin levels will be high and leptin levels will be low. When you have eaten a meal, your leptin levels will be high, and ghrelin levels will be low. This is the standard way these hormones are designed to function.

However, the problem begins when there is chronic inflammation of the fat cells. Frequent eating and excess fat accumulation can lead to such inflammation. The more fat you have, the more leptin there will be. Your fat cells keep releasing leptin and hence you shouldn't feel hungry at all or should feel satiated most of the time. Ideally, the answer will be yes. You should feel less hungry, more satisfied, and never have cravings for food. However, this doesn't happen thanks to the problem called leptin resistance caused by chronic inflammation in the fat cells.

In the case of obese people, the leptin levels are generally high. However, the hypothalamus of the brain stops registering these signals due to the unusually high levels of leptin all the time. This creates a severe problem. Your body keeps releasing the leptin hormone, but your brain doesn't recognize them. When an obese person is hungry, the change in the levels of the hunger hormone 'ghrelin' is also low. It is neither very high nor very low before or after eating. This also starts happening with the satiety hormone 'leptin.' In that case, an obese person will neither feel very hungry nor satisfied. There will always be a craving. This starts a vicious cycle of food consumption.

Feelings of hunger and fullness in an obese person are not the natural and appropriate responses of the body. The obese can perceive hunger when they see food and may never really get truly satisfied with the food. In this way, the quantity of ideal food consumption can never be a consideration for them. Such people will always have an irresistible craving for food and insatiable hunger. They will feel hungry in short bursts and food will always look like an irresistible option to them. However, this hunger is not driven by a requirement of their body, but a malfunction. The word 'malfunction' is key here.

We have understood that the obese person's response to food is not appropriate and it leads to more weight gain. We also know that their weight is also mostly responsible for it. Therefore, the repair of the system will also come from regulating these hormones.

Intermittent fasting can play a significant role in regulating the leptin hormone. You must make it clear in your mind that leptin is the master hormone for fat regulation in your body. It tells your body that the fat stores are abundant and therefore it should slow down the consumption of food. If the brain stops registering this signal, the fat stores will keep increasing. Chronic inflammation in the fat cells will drag you to that point. Overexposure of any particular hormone to the brain is responsible for the problem. If your body keeps releasing hormones all the time, the responsiveness of the brain to that hormone will decrease. The same happens with leptin too in the case of chronic inflammation.

Intermittent fasting helps you in normalizing the leptin release function. When your body remains in a fasted state for an extended period, it stops releasing the leptin hormone. During intermittent fasting, the release of leptin hormone slows down. Therefore, the leptin resistance starts to go down. Your sensitivity to leptin hormone improves, and you can feel satisfied more easily.

Leptin hormone regulation is essential for your fat burning process. As you know, it is a master hormone for fat regulation; it also controls the release of thyroid hormones. The thyroid hormones are the primary metabolic hormones. They increase metabolic functions and speed up burning of fat stores. If your body becomes resistant to leptin release, it will also have a slow metabolic function. Improved leptin sensitivity will mean that your metabolic rate will be high and you'll be able to burn fat more effectively. This is the way it should work.

You eat food, and your body starts releasing the leptin hormone to indicate fullness. The increase in the leptin triggers the thyroid hormones to step up metabolism to increase the fat burning process. However, the opposite happens in the case of obese people. Your leptin levels generally remain high, and other organs become resistant to it. Your metabolism stays slow, and you never achieve full satiety. Your brain also starts responding negatively. Instead of recognizing that your energy stores are full and sending signals to stop eating, your brain feels that you are starving. It sends messages to eat more and slows down the metabolic functions to conserve energy. Your capacity to burn fat drops drastically and your intake increases.

Improving leptin sensitivity is very important. It cannot be done until there is a constant focus on the reduction of your fat stores. Intermittent fasting can help in improving this issue.

Intermittent fasting helps in improving leptin sensitivity by normalizing leptin release. It also helps in curing the chronic inflammation in your fat cells. Your thyroid function also improves with the normalization of leptin release, and this speeds up the metabolic rate.

It becomes more natural and easy for your body to burn fat and to remain satiated for longer. After eating a meal once, you will feel satiety for longer. This puts an end to an incessant craving for food. Your ghrelin levels are also regulated, and HGH gets a considerable boost. Your metabolic rate also increases and you can lose overall weight fast.

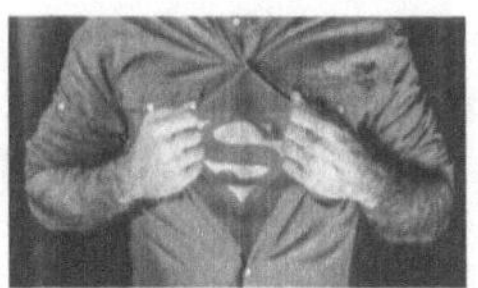

7

How it Boosts the Production of HGH, The Most Important Fat Burning Hormone

IN THE PAST FEW YEARS, the focus of the weight loss and wellness industry centralized towards one specific hormone, the Human Growth Hormone (HGH). This is an amazingly powerful performance-enhancing hormone.

This hormone accelerates fat loss like no other hormone.

- It helps in building muscle which explains the high focus of the bodybuilding industry towards it
- This hormone fills you with energy. You feel more lively, energetic and agile
- It has powerful anti-aging effects, and it promotes longevity
- The complete healing, growth, and repair function of your body gets a significant boost from this hormone

These are some of the reasons the HGH craze has emerged. However, after a certain age, our body slows down the production of this amazingly helpful hormone. The output of HGH is high in childhood as those are the formative years. Your body is growing fast, and it needs to build muscles and bones. The production of HGH is at its peak during puberty, but from there onwards, its output goes downhill. Our body still produces HGH but in small bursts and only in the right conditions. This hormone has such a substantial impact on growth, longevity, and aging that it's the reason people still want it in large quantities. This has led to the invention of synthetic HGH.

People are going left, right, and center to get synthetic HGH so that they can enhance their performance in competitive sports or reverse the signs of aging. The strong impact of HGH on athletes is a reason its use is banned in all competitive sports. Apart from the legal restriction, there are medical constraints too that require consideration. The natural HGH produced by our body has a unique structure. The synthetic HGH boasts of copying that structure, but that is far from being the truth. It will always remain a poor copy as our body has a very different way of functioning. The synthetic HGH boosts your performance for sure, but that enhancement doesn't come without side effects. People taking synthetic HGH can have joint pain, fluid retention, carpal tunnel syndrome, diabetes, heart diseases, and cancer. Because of these concerns, the use of synthetic HGH is prohibited in the US. However, the benefits of this hormone still lure people into taking the risk. In the year 2002 alone, around 100,000 people in the US received HGH illegally. The craze has been on a steady rise among teenagers too. A confidential survey conducted by Partnership for Drug-Free Kids revealed that the percentage of kids taking synthetic HGH doubled in one year from 2012-13. In 2011, 5 percent of teenagers were found to be taking synthetic HGH, and that figure reached 11 percent in the year 2013. This is an alarming number. However, considering the performance enhancing, fat burning, and anti-aging effects, people are ready to take the risk.

However, there is no need to take this risk when your body can still produce HGH if appropriately conditioned. The pituitary gland in our body produces HGH. This gland releases HGH in short bursts in special conditions.

The three most favorable conditions for HGH production are:

- When you are sleeping
- When you are doing high-intensity exercise
- When you are in trauma

However, there is a catch. Your body cannot produce HGH if there is a presence of insulin in your blood. Insulin blocks the production of HGH completely. If you have insulin resistance, then the situation gets even worse as the insulin levels in your blood remain consistently high. This inhibits the growth of HGH even more. One hormone that promotes the growth of HGH is ghrelin, the hunger hormone.

This is where intermittent fasting helps you. When you are following an intermittent fasting routine, you remain in a fasted state for an extended amount of time. Suppose you are following the OMAD routine and have your meal at 7 in the evening. Ideally, your body would release glucose from your last meal up to 8 hours. That means by 3 in the morning your insulin production would stop, as you wouldn't have any blood glucose. By this time, your hunger would have also picked up. Commonly, people are sleeping at this time of the night. It creates an ideal situation for the high growth of HGH. One study undertaken by the American College of Cardiology showed that the levels of HGH production increased up to 1300% in women and 2000% in men in this state.

Therefore, if your aim is fat burning, bodybuilding, better immunity, growth, anti-aging or longevity, intermittent fasting provides the best solution with the help of high HGH production.

However, the benefits don't end here. You can give a further boost to your HGH production by exercising in the fasted state. The longer you remain in the fasted state and exercise, the higher the production of HGH will be in your body.

Therefore, your weight loss and fat burning goal can be achieved with greater ease. This is among the prime reasons most of the bodybuilders have now started following OMAD routine for lean muscle gain and fat loss.

HGH is an essential hormone responsible for the healing, growth, and repair of every tissue in your body including the bones. Weight loss isn't the only benefit you'll get by high HGH production, as it will also boost your libido. Additionally, it improves your immune system and fills you with energy.

Intake of synthetic hormones for other than medical purposes is not only illegal but dangerous too. If you are following the OMAD routine, then you will never feel the need for synthetic HGH. The HGH produced naturally in your body is very helpful and effective. Your metabolism will surge, and you will be able to reduce your belly fat much faster than you can imagine. This is one of the primary reasons OMAD routine has become so popular. It strikes the belly fat where it hurts the most. It brings a positive change to your health biomarkers and makes you healthy.

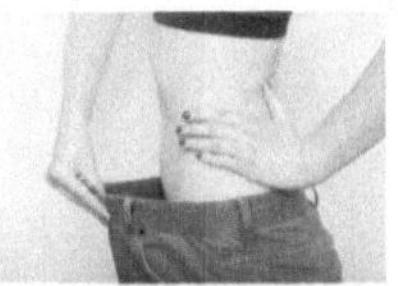

8

How it Boosts Your Metabolism

OBESITY IS A METABOLIC DYSFUNCTION. This term means that your calorie burning mechanism malfunctions and you are not able to burn as many calories as you consume. This is a problem state. The extra calories that you store daily are stored as fat, and you accumulate belly fat and weight.

The process is simple. Whenever you eat anything, the processed energy releases into your bloodstream in the form of glucose. The glucose is very easy to use as is it is a direct energy source. Our cells can use it in that form itself. The pancreas detects high levels of glucose, and it releases insulin to transport that glucose to the cells. Insulin acts as the power broker here. However, when you are consuming more energy than you can use instantly, it is initially stored as glycogen. Your liver and muscles store this as a backup source of energy and use it when you do not have a readily available supply of glycogen. However, if there is still excess energy, then the insulin deposits the surplus as fat in your abdominal tissues as visceral fat.

It should be clear that glucose is the preferred fuel of the body. As long as there is a supply of glucose in your blood, your body won't think of burning any other kind of fuel. This becomes a problem when you are frequently eating. Your body has a ready supply of glucose after short intervals. Even if you are on a calorie-restricted diet, your body keeps getting glucose spikes at regular intervals, and that prevents fat burning. Frequent meals also send a message to your body that it has an abundant supply of energy and it doesn't need to burn the fat reserves. This is among the primary reasons you are unable to burn excess fat even after being on a calorie-restricted diet.

The OMAD routine gives you an easy way out of this. Your blood sugar levels remain low. Your body takes around 12 hours to burn all the glucose in the blood and the glycogen stored in the liver. Once this reserve is depleted, it has no other option than to burn your fat reserves for energy. Hence, your body starts using the fat reserves and your belly fat burns. Intermittent fasting has a powerful impact on the improvement of your metabolic function.

Intermittent fasting leads to hormonal changes that ensure that insulin sensitivity improves. Higher insulin sensitivity improves your metabolic function. It leads to an increase in the growth of two important fat burning hormones. HGH and Norepinephrine. The whole process speeds up the fat burning, and you lose weight very quickly. Various studies have found that you can lose 3-8% weight over a period of 3-24 weeks on intermittent fasting. These studies have also concluded that you can also lose 4-7% of your waist circumference by intermittent fasting. Your overall health biomarkers improve, and you lose more body fat and less muscle mass. Several studies have also demonstrated that your metabolism increases up to 14 percent during fasts. This is a clear indicator that you can improve your metabolic function by intermittent fasting, burn your fat and experience weight loss.

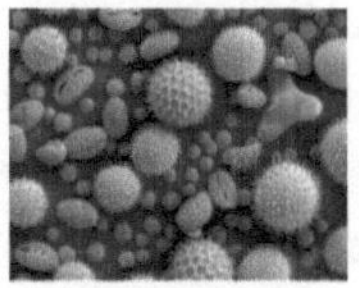

9

How it Helps in Curing Chronic Inflammation

CHRONIC INFLAMMATION IS a significant problem these days. Inflammation, in general, is a positive reaction of your body to any infection, disease, or germ attack. It starts the repair procedure and tries to heal your body. Nevertheless, an excess of anything is dangerous, and prolonged inflammation is very dangerous. When you have inflammation in any area of your body, it starts to affect your system negatively. In place of curing your body, it starts bringing it down. When an inflammation stays for too long, it is termed as chronic inflammation.

The thing that makes chronic inflammation more serious is the fact that usually, it is very low lying. It means that it's possible that you have chronic inflammation in any part of your body and you may remain oblivious to it for too long. This also means that it will keep affecting the proper functioning of your body, but you won't do anything for it, as there will be no apparent sign. It works like a slow poison. Obesity is also the result of one type of chronic inflammation; inflammation of the fat cells.

As previously discussed, fat cells release a hunger-suppressing hormone called leptin which makes you feel full and satisfied.

The controlled release of this hormone is essential for maintaining a healthy body. However, problems arise when there is chronic inflammation of the fat cells. This inflammation can be caused by some things like eating inflammatory food or frequent eating at short intervals. When your fat cells get inflamed, their leptin release function gets unregulated. Your fat cells continuously release the leptin hormone in small quantities all the time. This will make your body unresponsive to the signals it is designed to send. It will result in overeating and imbalance in your thyroid secretion as well, and these hormones have a direct relationship. Most people remain unaware of this fact and hence do nothing about it. When there is inflammation in your fat cells, suppressing the craving for food will be difficult for you. You will feel the need to eat more frequently, and that will cause weight gain. It will form a vicious cycle, and you will keep on putting on lots of weight.

The best way to heal such chronic inflammation is to avoid foods that cause inflammation and practice intermittent fasting. Anti-inflammatory foods will help soothe the causes of inflammation and give your body the ability to recover. Intermittent fasting, on the other hand, will give your body the time to recuperate. Regular intake of food keeps the leptin release constant and creates leptin resistance in your body. While you are on intermittent fasts, your body gets the time to recover from this resistance. Anti-inflammatory foods and intermittent fasting is the best combination to beat chronic inflammation.

Obesity is a condition that occurs due to a combination of several factors. If you try to overcome it by treating any one issue, the other factors will keep pulling you back. Taking a comprehensive approach that presents an answer to most of those issues is the best resort.

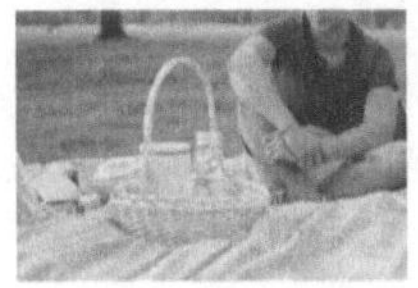

10

Following the OMAD Routine

WE HAVE DISCUSSED at length the things OMAD routine can do for you. It can bring a holistic change in your life and make you look and feel a lot better. You understand that you'll feel much healthier and comfortable in your skin. Although this all sounds good, remaining hungry for an extended period still seems a little intimidating.

If you are worried about being hungry for an extended period, then you need to hold your horses a bit. Suddenly starting the OMAD routine is neither required nor suggested. Switching to long fasting hours all at once isn't recommended. Your body has been running on quick, cheap energy provided by carbohydrates. To burn fat and remain energetic, your body will need to get 'Keto-Adapted.' This process takes time and patience. If you try to rush this process of extended fasting, then there are chances that your body will lose control and may start munching on your muscles too. Your blood sugar can also get low, and that isn't healthy either. You must make a slow transition. You will have to train yourself to remain without food, slowly and gradually.

Once your body gets comfortable with one level of fasting, only then you should move to the next level.

3 Meals a Day without Snacking in-between

At first, you should start training your body to stay on three meals a day. This means you can have breakfast, lunch, and dinner at usual timings. However, you must not consume anything else in the day. There should be no snacks or munching during the day besides those three meals. This isn't a fasting routine as the gap between the meals will be 4-5 hours. However, this is a good and healthy start, as gives your body time to assimilate. You can follow this routine until you no longer feel hungry between meals. The OMAD routine is a discipline. Every discipline needs training and patience. It is a process that needs to be followed with consistency. If you try to rush the process, then you may lose control midway. Therefore, it is vital that you first distance yourself from the extra snacking you have been doing. This will do two things for you. First, it will remove the empty calories you have been eating during the snack time. Secondly, it will train you to stay away from unnecessary indulgences.

Switching to the 16:8 Intermittent Fasting Routine

Once you are comfortable with not having anything in between the meals, you should reduce the number of hours in which you have those meals. This means, you can still have three meals a day, but you should reduce the gap between breakfast and dinner. Suppose that you previously had breakfast at 8 in the morning and dinner at 9 in the evening then this gave you a 13-hour eating window. You should start working on reducing this eating window. You can try shifting any one meal or both the meals a bit. You can have your breakfast at 11 in the morning and dinner at 7 in the evening. This brings down your eating window to 8 hours. You can try any combination as per your comfort. The only goal should be to minimize the eating window to 8 hours. This gives you a 16-hour fasting window. This should be the first intermittent routine you follow. This routine is called the 16:8 intermittent fasting routine. It also gives you some weight loss benefits, and it is easy to follow.

You'll find that you can follow this routine quite effortlessly. Let's examine the situation. An average person sleeps from 8-9 hours at night. Doctors all around the globe unanimously advise people to eat their last meal of the day 3-4 hours before going to sleep. Typically, you don't start eating as soon as you wake up. People have their breakfast 2-3 hours after they wake up. Even if you make small adjustments to your routine, following the 16:8 intermittent fasting routine would be a cakewalk for you.

This is a very powerful routine. It will give you most of the benefits of intermittent fasting, and you wouldn't have to compromise on anything. In the 8-hour eating window, you can eat almost anything. This is the first leg of intermittent fasting.

Important Fact

For all those folks who are trying to rush this process, please take a minute. Your body is an efficient machine, but it still runs like a machine. It has been running your body on a particular fuel, carbohydrates. Intermittent fasting is going to push your body to burn fat for fuel. Although fat is a cleaner and better fuel, your body isn't adapted to burn it in the beginning. This is why a slow transition so important. The process of burning fat is called ketosis. Your body can take 3 days to 6 weeks to switch to ketosis and therefore, rushing the process can prove to be counterproductive because it leaves you with no fuel at all during the transition.

Switching to the 20:4 Intermittent Fasting Routine

Once you are comfortable with the 16:8 fasting routine, only then should you move ahead. You should practice each method until you get accustomed to it. Never rush this process, your body needs to learn to sustain on the limited supply of blood glucose. Lack of this training will lead to 'Adrenaline Stress' in your body. You can start feeling lightheadedness, tired, thirsty, weak, and many other similar problems. These are all hypoglycemic symptoms. This means that your body suddenly goes low on blood sugar. This can lead to irritability and a strong craving for food. It is an undesirable condition. Earlier, frequent snacks and meals kept your body supplied with blood glucose. It has caused great damage to your body, but your body has been accustomed to it. Switching the routine too quickly will be equally harmful, and that's why a slow transition is suggested.

Once your body gets used to the 16:8 intermittent fasting routine, you should try narrowing your eating window once again. Once you have assimilated to an 8-hour eating window, start decreasing that eating window by an hour. Meaning, you can move to a 7-hour eating window. Once comfortable with that new fasting window, then bring it down to 6, and so on.

At first, try to eliminate one complete meal from your routine. You can do this by shifting your breakfast to the lunchtime. Bringing your eating window to 4 hours should be your ultimate goal here.

In this, you will fast for 20 hours and have all your meals in the 4-hour eating window. As the eating window decreases, you will find it difficult to eat three meals. Learning to have two healthy meals in this period is the best. You can eat the things you like in this window in any quantity. Intermittent fasting isn't a dieting routine. It focuses on burning the fat stores in your body. Incidentally, after 20 hours of fasting, your capacity to eat food will go down. You may feel very hungry in the beginning, but you wouldn't be able to eat food in a large quantity. The feeling of fullness will come very fast. This is a challenging routine to which to adapt. Your body will take some time to get used to this phase. However, this routine will return maximum weight loss benefits.

The 4-hour eating window is a minimal period. It is tough to have two full meals in this period, and you will end up with one fulfilling meal of the day. This is the One Meal a Day (OMAD) routine that should be your ultimate goal.

The OMAD routine is healthy and helps you burn fat fast and gain lean muscles. The popular misconception that you'll become weak and lose muscles is flat wrong. The fact that this is one of the most popular methods of the bodybuilding community should clear your doubts. Bodybuilders heavily rely on this routine for shedding extra body fat and gaining muscle mass.

Your body will start running on fat for fuel and become more efficient and energetic. The OMAD routine will also bring extra benefits like autophagy, which is an internal repair mechanism. The toxic waste in your body will be eliminated, and you will get additional benefits like increased growth and anti-aging too.

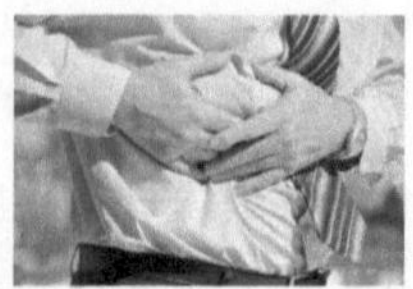

11

Coping with OMAD Diet

THERE IS no doubt that OMAD is a strict routine for many. People generally do not have much difficulty adjusting to the 16:8 phase as it works with the natural flow of life. However, when you are living on a single meal a day, things may be tough initially. The critical thing to remember is that your nutrition is paramount.

You must plan your meal wisely. Your one meal of the day should have a healthy combination of all the macro-nutrients and micro-nutrients. If you are thinking of surviving on the OMAD routine with junk food, then it will be an exercise in futility. You are kidding yourself and preparing a recipe for disaster.

Your meal should contain healthy fats, minerals, vitamins, protein, and energy. It should be a nutritious meal, and because you need to have all of it in one go, it should be tasty. The best thing about the OMAD routine is that it doesn't put a cap on the things you can eat and the things you can't. You are free to eat the stuff you like as long as it is healthy. You should utilize this opportunity to fill yourself with nutritious food.

People struggle to eat a lot in one go. However, as you start following the routine your capacity to eat more in a single meal expands. You won't feel underfed as you move along the way.

You can take mineral and vital supplements as you like. B Vitamins and Potassium supplements are especially beneficial. They help you overcome mineral and vitamin deficiencies. However, your focus should remain on taking a nutritious diet and make the most of it from this one meal.

Although you are not allowed to consume extra calories during the fasting period, you can drink non-caloric beverages like unsweetened fresh limewater, black coffee, and tea without sugar and milk. Green tea is also an excellent antioxidant and healthy beverage that you can take in the fasting window. However, the key is not to overdo these beverages. Tea and coffee will also help in suppressing your hunger and refreshing your mood.

You can drink water whenever you feel hungry. Taking water with fresh lime, and a dash of salt will help you avoid dehydration and strain. It will also assist you in suppressing hunger.

One meal a day may look a tall order initially, but once you start practicing it, you wouldn't feel the pressure. The slow transition and benefits it brings with itself will override all your inhibitions and apprehensions.

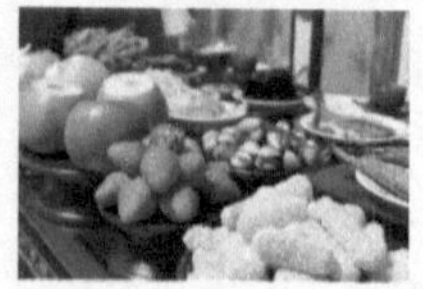

12

Preparing for Special Occasions or
Cheat Days

THE CONCEPT of the OMAD routine is excellent, and it has tremendous benefits. However, as the proverb rightly says, "All work and no play makes Jack a dull boy," following the OMAD routine regularly can take the fun out of it. We are social beings, and hence, we all have engagements where putting a restraint on food becomes difficult. Should you come home with a guilty conscience on those days? Of course not!

Cheat days play a helpful role in intermittent fasting. They give your body a chance to recuperate from the positive stress intermittent fasting has been exerting on your body. Your body gets the time to recover. The cheat days come as a reward and fill you with positivity, hope, and anticipation. Therefore, you must have cheat days on your schedule while following the OMAD routine.

The cheat days also play a unique role in your health. They help your body in resetting itself and making adjustments. They are the filler days. One thing to remember while having a cheat day is that you can't overdo it. The day after the cheat day you must return to the One Meal a Day routine. You can't have many cheats in a week or month, as that will also defeat the purpose.

However, you can have a cheat day on whichever day you like. So, if there is any special occasion on which you want to splurge, then take a break and enjoy the moment. Having the cheat days now and then will have a positive impact on your health too.

On the cheat days, there should be no restrictions on the number of meals you can eat. You will be free to eat anything you like and any number of meals you want. This will be your buffer day. Let yourself loose. Do not fret about the number of calories you are going to consume or the amount of time you need to give between your meals. This day should be for indulgence.

THE FIVE KEY Advantages of Having Cheat Days

Your Body Gets a Chance to Experience the Change and Make Adjustments

Change is essential in life. It breaks the monotonous nature of the routine and brings a freshness. When you take cheat days, your body shifts to the usual routine. It gets to experience the best of both the worlds. The cheat days helps your body in relaxing and takes off the strain. You get to eat without restriction, and your body makes an extra effort to accommodate that change. This keeps your system up and running. Following an OMAD routine puts your body in a specific routine. Your body starts working according to that routine, and its efficiency goes down with time. The cheat days shake off that routine. Your body starts showing better results from the OMAD routine. Hence, cheat days are surprisingly beneficial.

Your Body and Mind Get Relief from the Strain of Fasting

Fasting puts a healthy strain on your heart and the adrenal gland. Although this strain is training your body and does wonderful things, yet excess of even good things can be bad. Cheat days help your body in relaxing. You do not have to watch your diet or wait for long hours to eat. This relaxes your organs and relieves the stress. It is a very positive exercise. You will feel rejuvenated the next day and hence, it will become easier to begin the OMAD routine the next day. Also, but occasional breaks from the OMAD routine serve as a reward for all the effort you are putting in.

Your Insulin Sensitivity Improves

People with insulin resistance have an added advantage with the cheat days. These days help your pancreas to work more and adjust to the normal changes. Insulin resistance puts extra strain on the pancreas. OMAD routine limits the insulin secretion, as the blood glucose remains typically low. However, these cheat days help your body in testing the function of the pancreas and give your body a chance to check the insulin acceptance. This provides a significant boost to your insulin sensitivity. Having cheat days once in a week or fortnightly if your BMI is too high will help you a lot.

You Get a Chance to Relearn Healthy Eating

You get a chance to splurge on the cheat days. There is no restriction. However, a routine of eating only one meal a day restricts your eating habits a lot. These cheat days help you in returning to the full meal schedule. You get a chance to appreciate the things you have learned in the regimen and recognize the change in your diet. You get a free chance to eat anything you like, but you'll observe that your selection of food has become restrictive.

Nevertheless, there is no need to limit yourself to only a few items. You can eat even those things that you generally avoid on the routine days. This will also help in satisfying your cravings.

Cheat Days Help in Adjusting the High Energy Demands

One meal a day gives you a small eating window. Not only does it unintentionally restrict the number of calories you eat in a day, but it also limits the number of nutrients. Splurge days give you a chance to eat a variety of food items. Different kinds of foods have a variety of trace minerals that are important to us. This helps in preventing nutrient deficiency. You get many nutrients. On splurge days, you can eat excess calories. This is good for you, as in general, you'll be consuming fewer calories. It also helps you in feeling better and motivated. Your body will also learn to adjust the extra calories in routine.

There are only two important things to remember with cheat days. First, you should never take consecutive cheat days. There should be fasting days between the cheat days. This helps your body in maintaining the balance, and your control also remains intact. Second, always try to plan your cheat days around special events so that you can enjoy those days with your friends and family without guilt.

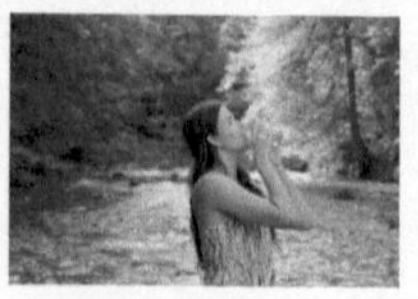

Boost the Benefits of OMAD Routine with Occasional Extended Water Fasting

STUDIES HAVE REPEATEDLY DEMONSTRATED the advantages of fasting. The benefits of fasting far outweigh the efforts required for fasting. It accelerates your weight loss efforts, cleanses, boosts anti-aging, and promotes longevity among other good things. Fasting gives our body a chance to recover and repair. If there is one thing that gives a boost to the effects of fasting, then it is water fasting.

Water fasting, as the name suggests, is the process of keeping the fast by only consuming water. You go without eating anything at all for extended periods. This type of fasting can extend from 24 to 72 hours safely. People under supervision can keep water fasts for even longer and enjoy better health.

One thing is crucial to understand: that you shouldn't undertake long water fasts without consulting a medical doctor. If you suffer from chronic illness, or you are on any medication, it becomes all the more important. Water fasting is serious business. It will lead to the proper cleansing and detoxification of your system. Doing it without consulting a physician can cause complications for people on medication.

Water fasting, if done correctly, can do amazing things to your body. It revitalizes your whole system. One powerful process that kicks in with water fasts is *autophagy*. This is the internal repair and maintenance mechanism. Your body starts producing lots of stem cells that lead to regeneration of lost cells and muscles.

Water fasting is a powerful tool that can give you a head start for a healthy life. If you were already following the OMAD routine, then fasting won't be a problem for you. Water fasting will lead to relaxation of your gut.

Our whole body is a complex mechanism. It works day-in and day-out tirelessly. However, one part of your body never gets rest, and that's your gut. It is always at work digesting food and replenishing the good gut bacteria. During water fasting, this system enjoys a much-needed respite. Therefore, after the water fasting your digestion mechanism improves considerably.

One critical thing that you must always remember while water fasting is that you shouldn't end your water fast in a haphazard manner. The progression to eating must always be slow and organized. Not doing so can be dangerous as your body takes time to adjust to the assault of food items.

You must plan carefully before and after the water fast. Your body is going to cleanse itself during the water fast, and you must create a natural environment for that.

Before a Water Fast

When you plan to begin your water fast, it is crucial that you go easy on food. Eating difficult-to-digest food items a few days before a water fast can be a bad idea. You will want your gut to relax. Try to go on a vegetable and fruit diet at least three days before you begin your water fast. These items are easy to digest, and your system will be able to clear them quickly. Meat and greasy food are difficult to clean as it gets stuck, and therefore consuming a lot of meat and fatty stuff will not be a great idea.

During the Water Fast

Water fasting should always be done on days when you can give your body time to relax. Weekends or long vacations are an excellent opportunity for water fasts. On these days, your focus shouldn't be on straining your body. You can give heavy exercise or strenuous activity a break on these days. The first day should be easy as you'll be spending the energy of the food consumed the previous day. The second day will jump-start fat burning, as you will be low on energy and your body will also start cleansing. Relaxing during this time is very helpful. On the third day, your body will have adapted to the fat burning, and you may feel the surge of energy. There may not be any craving for food at all. You can break your fast at the end of the third day with vegetable juice or broth.

Ending the Water Fast

Stopping the water fast is a critical part. Your body has been in a relaxing mode. Your gut is clean and relaxed. If you start eating whole grains or hard vegetables on the first day of breaking your water fast, your gut may revolt. You will want to avoid that unpleasant scenario. Always end your water fast slowly and gradually. Start by drinking vegetable juice or broth as the first meal to break your fast. It replenishes your system and doesn't strain it. Broth gives you the nutrients and has less sugar. Therefore, there is a very low risk of high blood sugar. You can also take vegetable soup later in the day to get energy. On the second day, you can eat fruit juice or smoothies too if you do not have problems like diabetes. You should begin slowly and take only soft or mashed food that is easy to digest. Give your gut time to adapt, and move to a solid diet and raw vegetables slowly.

The progression is important because if you start splurging right after your water fast, then the whole effort goes down the drain.

Water fasting has immense benefits, but it does put a bit of strain on your body. Therefore, it is essential to take all the necessary precautions. If you do it correctly under supervision, then it can give you great health benefits. The key to water fasting is control. If you are in the habit of bingeing after fasts, then water fasting is not for you.

Water fasting will cleanse your cells and lead to weight loss. Your body will get the time it needs to get off the empty calories and burn fat reserves.

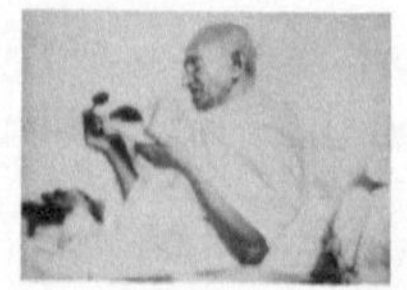

How Long to Do Water Fasting

THE DURATION of water fasting would vary from person to person. A healthy person who isn't on medication or not suffering from any chronic illness can do longer fasts. It would depend upon the endurance of the person and specific needs. There is no definitive formula for that.

However, if you are following an OMAD routine, then doing water fasting should only be treated as a cleansing exercise. Water fasting up to 3 days should serve the purpose well for you. However, it is not mandatory to be on water fasting for three days at a stretch.

Going slow is the best policy while dealing with any fasting. You should always begin with one-day fasting and increase the duration over a period.

People water fast for longer durations too. Some people water fast over a period of 40 days under strict medical supervision. However, it is not necessary for people on an OMAD routine, as they need water fasting only for cleansing the body and triggering autophagy. The weight loss benefits will come with the

OMAD routine alone, and there is very little chance that you'll be carrying water weight.

You can continue with your OMAD routine and enjoy 'cheat days' after short intervals as well. You should also take care to drink plenty of water and begin your water fast correctly.

The frequency of water fasting shouldn't be too often. You can do water fasting once every three months and then more often, to once a month. Do not try to overdo water fasting and stick to your OMAD routine as much as possible.

Water fasting should only be used as an occasional tool and not your primary mode. You are not going to do water fasting for weight loss but instead for better healing and cleansing. Do not try to mix both these concepts.

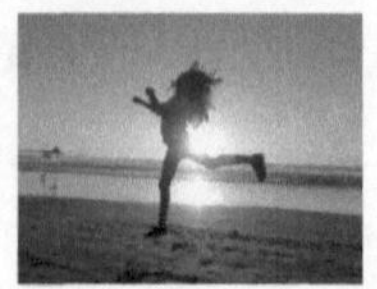

15

Trigger Autophagy for Cellular Healing

AUTOPHAGY IS a much talked about phenomenon these days. This process has been in discussion since 1960, but recently, a Japanese scientist named Yoshinori Ohsumi enlightened the scientific community on the process and won the Nobel Prize in 2016 for his detailed research on the effects of autophagy on our bodies.

Simply put, autophagy is the ability of our body to clean itself of all the waste and toxic material. We have all heard about the metabolic processes. We know that our metabolism helps us in burning fat and keeps our body going. However, the details of the process are usually overlooked. Metabolism is a balance of two kinds of antagonistic processes in our body, anabolism, and catabolism. Anabolism is the process of synthesizing molecules and building structures while catabolism breaks down molecules and structures. Autophagy is a catabolic process of breaking down the macromolecules within the cells.

Dr. Yoshinori discovered in his research that this process of autophagy has great potential of curing many diseases. Autophagy can not only lead to the cleansing of the cells but may also halt the progression of many diseases and induce anti-aging effects.

It is an astonishing process where the body can detect all the problems going on and weed out the cause of the issues on its own. The thing that makes it awesome is that fact that your body doesn't need your help at all in carrying out this process. This process is most active and productive when you are doing nothing at all. This may come as a surprise for most; however, this is the truth, plain and simple.

We all know that our bodies go through a lot in the ordinary course of life. We assault it with all kinds of inflammatory food items. Some diseases cause problems for our bodies. The pesticides, insecticides, sprays and other types of chemical waste get into our system. Then, there is a continuous process of cell building, degeneration, and regeneration. Our body produces a countless number of cells on an ongoing basis. All these things create waste. Our body produces mostly helpful items but it is a machine, and it also produces defective cells at times that can't be utilized. They remain as waste in the body.

Our body has the potential to clean itself. It can productively use all these waste materials. However, we never give it a chance.

Our body is a very efficient machine. In times of need, our body can use even the last shred of material in the body to keep itself alive. However, our continuous onslaught never gives it a chance. Autophagy is the chance our body needs. It can help in the disintegration of all the toxic waste and, in turn, produce new cells and energy. There is only one condition necessary for this process to work and that condition is a short supply of energy from external sources.

This means that our body can only begin autophagy on an extensive scale when it starts feeling the supply of energy from external sources has stopped. In that case, the body will go into survival mode and start burning all the waste inside itself to conserve energy and produce more. The prerequisite for this process is that you will have to stop the continuous supply of energy for a certain period.

Water fasting is the process that comes into play here. Water fasting restricts your calorie intake for a certain period and leaves your body scavenging for energy.

At the cellular level, our cells contain defective and damaged cell parts. There are intracellular pathogens that are useless and may be causing harm. Then, there are mis-folded proteins that have been misshaped and are of no use. All these things are of no use to your body and can be utilized. Autophagy strikes all these at first.

Your cells have an enzyme called Lysosome, which works as the recycler. When you go on a prolonged fast, your body starts detecting that it is not getting any more energy. This activates the lysosomes, and they start recycling all this waste mentioned above and produces free fatty acids and amino acids. Both of these things are used for generating energy and remodeling cells.

Autophagy is a process that will stop all chronic inflammatory response in your body as it is using up energy. It will heal long illnesses that have been troubling you for years. Even patients with terminal diseases like cancer see tremendous improvements through this process because it stunts the growth of cancer cells. Autophagy will stop all the problem-causing processes in your body and will work towards conserving energy and producing new cells. The sole aim is to keep you going for longer.

Your body can eliminate all kinds of pathogens like fungi, molds, and bacteria. It will discard all the waste material from your body. This process is beneficial for your brain, heart, and immune system. Your immune system gets a substantial boost, as your body resists infections. The cell remodeling and new cell growth also bring wonderful anti-aging effects, and you'll look and feel better.

During water fasting, your body also produces stem cells in large quantities. The focus of your body at this time is to survive. It makes the best efforts to eradicate problems and make the system more secure.

Scientists have discovered that autophagy has a profound effect on the brain. It leads to the regeneration of cells that can reverse the effects of neurodegenerative disorders like Alzheimer's and Parkinson's. People with dementia and other such problems also get great benefits from this process. Your cognitive functions improve, and you can function better as a whole.

Autophagy also has a significant impact on your heart as well. It also leads to the regeneration of heart cells. If you are suffering from cardiovascular disorders, then this is your cue.

Overall, autophagy promotes longevity by improving your vital parameters. If you are suffering from problems like hypertension, heart disease, immunity disorders, chronic inflammation or other similar issues, then autophagy is your solution. When the process of autophagy begins your body starts releasing a chemical called Sirtuin. This chemical can stop the growth of most of the diseases in the body. People with many lifelong issues like rheumatoid arthritis, cancer, and diabetes begin the healing process.

However, autophagy cannot start on its own. It will not begin if you have a continuous supply of energy. If you keep eating and have high levels of insulin, then autophagy cannot occur. Insulin is at the heart of any problem. Yes, we are going there again!

Insulin resistance is a major problem for our body. When there is much insulin in your body, and it is not working correctly, it leads to the accumulation of much waste. It causes oxidative stress and generates amyloid deposits.

Autophagy has the potential to undo these issues. It can clear your system. It can purge all the waste accumulated in your body and make it efficient and fully functional.

Two things that lead to autophagy are water fasting and intermittent fasting.

During the water fasts, you completely stop the consumption of calories in any form and force your body to produce energy on its own. It generates energy by burning your fat stores. However, the presence of toxic waste would lead to inefficiency.

If you follow an OMAD routine, then your energy consumption would go down naturally. You'll also start burning fat deposits. Your body will be in a functional state of ketosis. If you water fast during this period, then autophagy will work excellently. You will have made the process easy.

Apart from fasting, more things help in the autophagy process such as:

Aerobic exercises like walking and yoga: These activities help in keeping the flow of energy smooth. You can get great benefits from autophagy if you exercise or do yoga. These aren't strenuous activities, and your body gets the right supply of oxygen.

Food items containing sulforaphane: This is a phytonutrient found in cruciferous vegetables. This helps in the process of the regeneration of damaged cells. If you have been eating vegetables containing sulforaphane, then regeneration becomes easier.

Vitamin D3 and B3: These two vitamins are beneficial in the process of autophagy. You should focus on eating things that are rich in both these vitamins.

Coffee: This beverage is also a good source of phytonutrients helpful in the regeneration of the nerve cells. However, you shouldn't overdo the use of coffee as too much of it can be counterproductive.

Green Tea: This is an herbal beverage, and it helps in the regeneration of the nerve cells.

Coconut: This tropic fruit is also perfect for people who want to boost the process of autophagy.

Water fasting is an easy way to trigger this fantastic process. It can make you healthier while you are on your way to extreme weight loss.

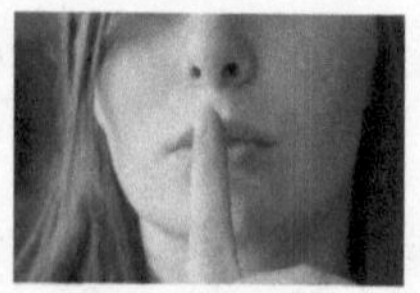

16

Do I Tell People I Am Fasting?

IF YOU ARE overweight or an obese person, then you know what it is to live in an unfit body. There are tons of problems within yourself, but that's not the end of it. With obesity also comes mocking, scorn, taunts, and fat shaming. People make rude comments and you with disdain. This can be more than enough heartbreak for a person already struggling with so much.

If you start telling people at the beginning that you are intermittent fasting or following an OMAD routine, you may become a target of derision and sarcasm. Avoid these people during the process. Our actions will speak for us.

The day you start losing weight, it will become evident to the world on its own. You won't need to tell anyone at all. Weight loss will come as a pleasant surprise to some and a shock to others. Talking about your routine, in the beginning, will only bring more sarcasm and should be avoided.

However, following a strict routine without confiding in anyone is also a difficult task. We need someone to talk to and listen to us.

Your family and very close friends who sympathize with your condition and feel for you are the best for this.

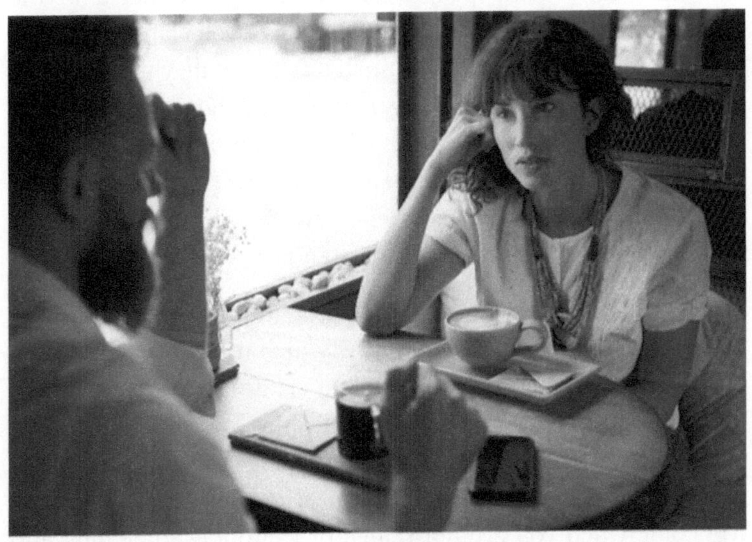

Disclosure to a select group of people is essential. Every addictive thing has withdrawal symptoms. Studies have found that sugar is eight times more addictive than cocaine. You will be drawing yourself away from added sugar, artificial sweeteners, fast food, binge eating, and more. In the beginning, there can and will be cravings. There should be people to help you when you are about to give up. There should be some people in a close-knit group to encourage you to continue when you want to give in to the temptation to eat. Therefore, confiding in some people is important.

Although confiding in a few people is recommended, the selection of those people should be wise.

You should look for the following qualities to identify the people with whom you can share the details of your OMAD routine:

Understanding. Extended periods of fasting can cause irritation and frustration at times. This usually happens more in the first couple of days when the body is craving for sugar and food. You must have some people who thoroughly understand the reason for such anger bouts. Confiding with your family, partner, or roommates is the best in such cases, as they become the biggest recipients of your anger outbursts. They will not only understand you and sympathize with you, but it will also prevent bitterness seeping into your relationships. Ultimately, when everything settles down, you will have people to support and share with you. Patience and understanding is the key here.

Open to Discussion. Weight loss is a gradual process. It won't occur overnight. If the people in whom you have confided start prompting such questions too often, it creates a feeling of failure. The self-doubt seeps in, which is unhealthy. You should discuss it with those people who are understanding and appreciate the process. A healthy discussion is critical in such cases. The time will come when you are not doing, or overdoing something and need to change your ways. If such people do not talk to you in these cases, then you will not be able to make suitable adjustments.

People with Keen Observation Skill. If you have people around who can keenly observe your routine and your progress, then it helps. They can guide you and correct if you are doing anything wrong. Confiding in people who are also following such methods or are willing to do so is also great. They'll watch you more closely, and you will be able to assess the success or short-comings easily.

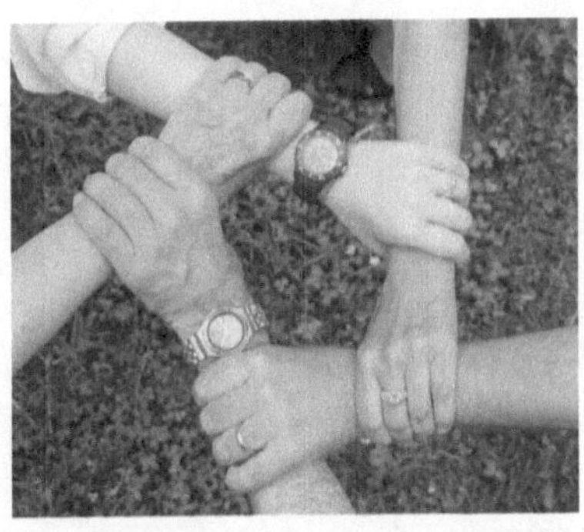

Respectful. Although a bit of frankness and truthfulness is helpful, it shouldn't be blunt. Honestly without tact is cruelty. People who gently tell the truth are always more useful than those who don't. People trying to lose weight are already going through too much. If they also need to face sarcasm from people around them, then it becomes difficult. Especially, those people who know about your efforts must comment respectfully.

Joining a Support Group

Support groups are great when it comes to getting away from any addiction whether it is drugs, alcohol or food. When you begin fasting, a lot is going inside your body and your head.

Many hormonal changes take place in your head. Your body starts switching the fuel mechanism and does the fine-tuning. Initially, your brain also goes into overdrive and starts sending you erratic signals to eat. Some people get a strong urge to eat, and the temptation to quit is powerful. Support groups help a lot at this stage.

Being with people suffering from the same condition and listening to them helps you in warding off temptation. You get strength from their stories and find them motivational. The success of other people in your support group will inspire you.

Support groups have likeminded people suffering from the same condition. You can seek strength in them when you feel weak or intimidated. You can find non-judgmental people who won't look you up and down before commenting.

However, you must always remember that the best support is going to come from you. Excess weight is a liability for you. It is stopping you from achieving the life you could have. It prohibits you from living the life you want. It has stolen the body in which you want to live proudly. You need to drive the excess weight out and get into shape. The biggest motivation has to come from you. Always stay positive and repeat affirmations whenever you feel weak or unmotivated. The OMAD routine is easy to follow, and the hunger pangs would be the least of your worries after the initial days have passed. You will lose weight very quickly, get into shape, and feel healthy.

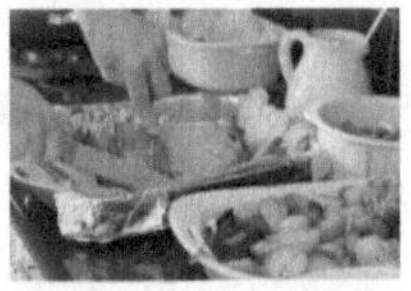

17

OMAD Routine and Keto Diet, A Match Made in Heaven

OVERBEARING fat is a big problem and a reality of the current American lifestyle. With the majority of the American population facing the obesity epidemic, we can't keep feigning ignorance. The OMAD routine presents an easy way to lose weight. It is sustainable and very effective. You will not only lose the temporary water weight but also actually burn the visceral fat for good.

A Ketogenic diet helps you with that. The Keto diet is the right way to lose fat. For beginners, the ketogenic diet is a high-fat, moderate protein, and low-carbohydrate diet. It shifts your body from burning carbohydrates to fat.

For all those people who are wondering, when they adopt an OMAD routine to burn body fat, why should they be eating more fat? There is an answer. However, for that, you will have to understand the mechanism by which our body uses energy.

We usually run our body on carbohydrate fuel. Most of the things we eat are high in carbohydrates. It is digested quickly and gives us glucose. Our liver can process it quickly and then our pancreas releases insulin to use up all that glucose. The extra glucose then gets converted into glycogen and fat. However, in this whole process, our body is only burning up carbohydrates and stops burning fat. This creates the entire problem of fat accumulation in the first place.

When you begin a keto diet, you deprive your body of carbohydrate fuel and force it to burn fat. The fat is a difficult fuel to burn but releases a high amount of energy. In the process, our body also starts burning its body fat to power itself, and then real fat loss occurs.

However, our body will not start burning fat until and unless the supply of carbohydrate fuel is completely shut off. Two very different kinds of mechanisms are required to burn these energy sources. Eventually, insulin is at the base of the whole problem.

When you are continuously eating high carbohydrate and abusing your system with frequent meals, insulin resistance begins.

You start facing a multitude of problems like:

- Belly Fat
- Hypertension
- Diabetes
- Fatigue
- Memory loss
- Lack of focus
- Anxiety
- Depression

Your body stops responding to high insulin secretion and develops insulin resistance. We have already discussed that insulin resistance leads to problems and fat gain is one among them.

One way to get over insulin resistance and increase insulin sensitivity is to lower blood sugar levels. This is what the keto diet does for you.

When you go on a keto diet during your OMAD routine, your blood sugar levels go down, and your body switches to burning the fat fuel in place of carbohydrate fuel. Lowering sugar intake is a critical requirement for this process to begin.

You can easily satisfy this condition by switching to a keto diet. However, there may be some initial difficulties with this process. Your body has been addicted to sugar. When you begin a low-carbohydrate diet, your blood sugar levels may drop.

You may face the following symptoms for a few days:

- Strong cravings
- Lightheadedness
- Hunger
- Fatigue
- Constipation

You won't have to worry too much about these symptoms as they are temporary and they will recede with time. There are easy ways to manage these symptoms.

You can ward off the initial problems by doing the following things:

Fatigue: B5 deficiency. You may feel fatigue in the beginning. You can easily overcome this fatigue by taking Vitamin B5 supplements.

Cramps: Potassium deficiency. Cramps and constipation is a common issue. However, most of this problem is due to potassium deficiency, and you can overcome it by consuming green vegetables. While you are on a keto diet, eat a lot of green vegetables. Cruciferous vegetables have lots of potassium, and they'll help you with these symptoms. They are very healthy and fulfill a vitamin and mineral deficiency.

Bloating: Bile Salts. Bloating is also a common problem encountered by people on a keto diet. An easy way to deal with this problem is to go slow on fats. People may start consuming too much fat at the very beginning. Understand that your body is going to make a switch. You will have to go slow on the fat. Take sea salt in place of table salt and increase its daily intake a bit. This will help you in overcoming the problems.

Sleep Issues: Calcium Magnesium deficiency. People start facing problems related to sleep. This can easily be managed by eating a lot of green vegetables. They contain a lot of calcium and magnesium, and your sleep would improve.

Decalcification: Take Lime. The keto diet and the OMAD routine lead to decalcification. Many calcium deposits that are clogging your system get cleaned. This may lead to the development of uric acid and kidney stones. The easy way to manage this problem is to increase the intake of lemon. Consume at least one lemon in a day or more. Drink fresh limewater or lemon or citrus fruits, but consuming lemon is essential. This will help in cleaning your system and help you avoid these problems.

One more problem people face while on the keto diet, and the OMAD routine is that they feel too stuffed. The reason behind this problem is overeating. You have a fewer number of meals in a day. You try to eat as much as you can. Although there is no calorie restriction in the OMAD routine, overeating can make you feel stuffed. Do not overeat. Your body will run fine on fat in the absence of caloric intake.

Some people find that their cholesterol levels increase while on a keto diet. There is no reason to get alarmed. This cholesterol is not the dietary cholesterol. When your body burns fat, it releases cholesterol and triglycerides. It uses them as fuel and therefore, the levels would be naturally higher in comparison to a typical state. However, cholesterol is not a bad thing. It is the building block of hormones and other beneficial things in your body. Your cholesterol levels will stabilize after some time, and you would start feeling great.

The important thing is to get off sugar. As long as you have readily available glucose fuel, even in small quantities, your body won't start burning fat. Your body takes around 72 hours to consume all the accessible energy stored in the form of glucose and glycogen. Once these sources are depleted, your body has no other option than to burn fat. You will not only lose water weight with the help of keto diet but will also lose belly fat. This means that over a period, your waist circumference will shrink and you will have a leaner body.

Some people feel that after a certain period they stop losing weight on a keto diet. There is a strong reason for that. Once your body loses the water weight and starts burning fat, your body also starts building muscle mass. Muscle is dense, more than fat. So you get thinner, while your weight may increase. This is a positive thing. The correct way to measure your progress on a keto diet is to measure your weight as well as waist circumference. Your weight may stop decreasing after a certain amount of time, but your waist circumference will keep shrinking.

The keto diet helps you lose weight and get a leaner and muscular frame. You become healthy and have an abundance of energy. You will feel better all day and get rid of many lifestyle disorders.

There are seven strong benefits of following a Keto Diet:

High Energy Levels. Fat fuel is the superior fuel for your body. It leaves no toxic waste and keeps your body running for long, which is why your body chooses to store it for contingency measures. This fuel can keep you running healthily for long even on a smaller diet.

Weight Loss. The keto diet speeds up your weight loss. This diet blocks your carbohydrate intake. You start running the body on fat. This helps in burning body fat. You will lose fat quickly and get a better figure. It is the best way to gain lean muscle mass.

Improved Memory. The keto diet gives you a ton of antioxidants. They help with your brain function. The hormonal levels also improve in your body which helps in neurological function. The OMAD routine along with a keto diet gives a boost to autophagy that improves memory and decreases neurodegenerative disorders.

Improves Mood. The fluctuating glucose levels on a carbohydrate meal can give you mood swings. This is not the case with the fat fuel. The fat fuel burns slowly but consistently and releases a high amount of energy. This keeps your mood stable, and you stop experiencing mood swings.

Cravings and Hunger Go Away. This is one of the best benefits of being on a Keto diet while following an OMAD routine. As your body keto-adapts, it stops having the cravings for sugar and hunger pangs. It has a steady source of energy, and you do not feel hunger for long. The people on longer fasts stop feeling hunger at all. Therefore, you can work with great focus, and your attention will be undivided.

Better Metabolism. The keto diet improves your metabolism. Your body burns fat more efficiently and yields excellent results.

Improves Insulin Resistance. Insulin may be a cause of

most of the health issues, but it is an essential hormone. Insulin resistance caused by disorderly food intake can lead to several problems. The **OMAD** routine and a keto diet help you in improving insulin dysfunction and restore insulin sensitivity. It is highly beneficial for you and will bring positive health effects.

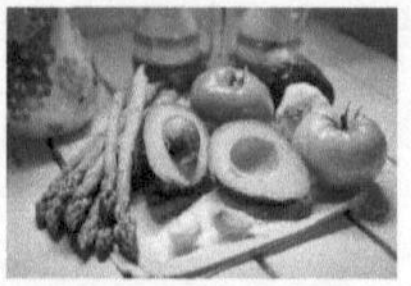

Things to Eat on a Keto Diet

YOUR KETO DIET should contain high fat and balanced protein. Almost 70% of the calories should come from fat, 20% of the calories should come from protein, 5% of the calories can come from vegetables, and the remaining 5% from carbohydrates.

Fats

This is merely an estimate. Although the fat brings the highest amount of calories, you shouldn't consume too much fat. Remember that fat is calorie dense and even a small amount of fat may have too many calories. The percentage of fat you can consume daily will have to be adjusted based on need. If you feel bloated for hours after eating, then you would need to go light on the fat. Lower the amount of fat you are eating, and that should work fine.

Proteins

The proteins constitute the second macro that you are going to consume. However, choose healthy protein and do not go overboard with it. You must also remember that protein shouldn't be the first thing that you consume in the morning as it can increase your blood sugar. You should also remember not to overeat protein, as overeating protein is easy. Not eating enough protein could have consequences as your body may start eating its muscles. Moderation is the key here.

Vegetables

Vegetables should make up only 5% of calories to a keto meal, but they are critical. You will be eating vegetables in the highest quantity as they do not add too many calories, but give you a lot of vitamins, minerals, and trace elements that are essential for your body. You shouldn't compromise on vegetables and must have at least 7 cups of vegetables every day. You can drink them as smoothies and vegetable salads. You should start your day with vegetables as you can eat them in large quantities without increasing calories or sugar. They will also reduce your appetite. Sprouts are also great as they also supply many phytonutrients.

Carbs

Consume carbohydrates only in minimal quantities. Their calorie contribution shouldn't be more than 5%.

Getting the right amount in the first go is difficult. You will have to make adjustments in the beginning to find the right fit.

You need to consume fats in high quantity. Be warned; not all fats are good for you. They may help you with your weight loss but may also cause deficiencies. Therefore, it is crucial that you include the right kind of fat in your diet.

Good Sources of Healthy Fat

Seafood and Fish. Seafood and especially the wild caught salmon, or fatty fishes are the best sources of healthy fat. They contain a high amount of Omega-3 fatty acid that has excellent anti-inflammatory properties.

Eggs and Chicken. Farm-raised chicken eggs are also a good source of fat. However, you must remember that you wouldn't get the same benefits from commercial eggs. The poultry chicken is treated with many antibiotics, and that reduces the nutritional content in the eggs. The same goes for chicken.

Grass Fed Meats. Meat that has been grass-fed and not grain fed is a good source of fat. You can include such fat in your diet. However, grain fed meat is not that helpful.

Nuts. Walnuts, almonds, macadamias and other such nuts are a good source of healthy fats.

Flax seeds. You can take these into your diet. However, the process of conversion of these into healthy fats and Omega-3 is complex. You cannot rely on them for providing sufficient fat and Omega-3.

Other fats that you might eat on a daily basis like peanut butter, sunflower oil, and other seed oils contain fat, but they lack in Omega-3 fatty acids. They have a high amount of Omega-6 fatty acids that aren't very healthy. If you rely solely on them for your fat intake, then there will be an imbalance of Omega-3 to Omega-6 in your body, and that's undesirable. Stick to butter, ghee, coconut oil, or macadamia nut oil as healthy choices.

The Key Items to Eat on a Keto Diet

Vitamin C. Your body suffers heavy damage while on a carbohydrate diet. High levels of sugar and insulin cause severe damage to your liver, kidneys, heart, and brain cells. Vitamin C is essential for the repair work. You must include a lot of Vitamin C rich food in your diet. Green bell pepper provides a generous source of vitamin C. There are other things too, like Sauerkraut, which is a good source of vitamin C. You must consume these items in good quantity. You get this vitamin from most of the green vegetables and lemon.

Omega-3 Fatty Acids. Omega-3 fatty acid is essential for heart health, and it also helps with inflammation. Wild-caught salmon and fatty fish are a rich source of Omega-3. You can also take virgin cod liver oil.

Vitamin B1. B Vitamins are essential for you. You get them from sunflower seeds, pork, and nutritional yeast. You must consume them in your diet.

Potassium and Magnesium. You need potassium and magnesium to run your body properly. Potassium deficiency can lead to fatigue and several other problems. You can easily get both these minerals from green vegetables. You must include many leafy vegetables in your diet. At least 7-8 cups of vegetable consumption are necessary to keep you healthy. Plants are low on calories, and therefore you can consume them in almost unlimited quantities.

Iodine. Iodine is another vital thing to include in your diet. You get iodine from seafood so you must try to include this in your diet.

Iron. It is an essential mineral, and you can get plenty of it by eating red meat or organ meat.

Phytonutrients. Phytonutrients are key to the functioning of your brain cells, and you must include them in your diet. You can get many phytonutrients from the sprouts. Broccoli sprouts are very rich in phytonutrients.

Eating the right foods will return the best results. The ketogenic diet is a process. Selecting the right things for your ketogenic diet will provide a boost to the process. Your body will be able to reduce fat while minimizing side effects.

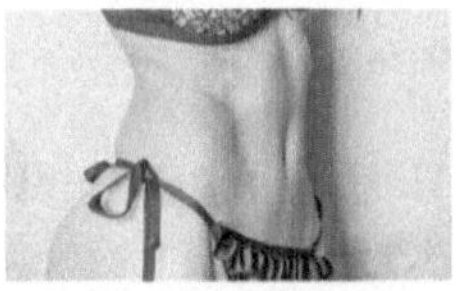

Benefits of OMAD Routine

THE OMAD ROUTINE brings a holistic change in your life. It is a comprehensive health package in itself. By practicing the OMAD routine, you not only ensure physical and mental, but spiritual well-being too. People all around the world of all races, classes, and weight groups are trying this amazing routine and get astounding results.

However, apart from all other benefits, this routine offers, the one that stands out from the rest is extreme weight loss. If your protruding belly and overbearing weight are becoming a reason for concern then, the OMAD routine can give you great relief. It will help you in shedding the extra pounds fast and in getting rid of the unpleasant looking tummy spare tire.

The problem with obesity is that people see it in the wrong light. Obese people will swear by anything that they'll start living a healthy life once they get rid of the weight. They fail to recognize that it is their unhealthy lifestyle that has caused this problem of obesity in the first place. The truth is, obesity is the symptom, not the cause of the problem. If they had followed a healthy lifestyle, there wouldn't have been the problem of obesity at all. You will have to treat the cause, and the effect will come on its own.

If you have a healthy body, then keeping it lean and fit will be comparatively easy. It is not due to the leaner stature, but due to the absence of health issues.

Let us consider some common issues any typical obese person under 40 years of age faces these days:

- Cardiovascular problems
- High Cholesterol
- High Blood Pressure
- Diabetes
- Liver Dysfunction
- Digestion Issues
- Metabolic Disorders
- Chronic Inflammation
- Fatigue
- Stress
- Anxiety
- Eating Disorders
- Acidity

These are the common disorders. If you test any random obese person, then the chances are high that at least, half of these diseases would surely be identified in that person. This is a disturbing scenario, and it is not going to improve on its own.

A fit and healthy person of the same age probably won't have even a couple of these issues. The reason is simple; obesity is a result of these problems. If you are not overweight or obese, then there is a higher likeliness that you won't have these complications too at such an early stage.

The saddest part is that these problems claim more than 500,000 preventable deaths in the US alone, every year. If you start following a healthy lifestyle, you can dodge most of these problems easily. It's as simple as that. There is a reason that most of these problems are called lifestyle disorders. Your poor lifestyle and eating habits can cause these problems.

The OMAD routine gives you an excellent opportunity to rectify all the mistakes that have led to obesity. If you are a healthy person and do not need to lose weight, then it can help you in efficiently maintaining your physique and gaining muscle and strength.

OMAD is a wonderful weight loss measure, but the benefits don't end at weight loss. As stated above, the OMAD routine improves your health biomarkers and makes you healthy. Weight loss is a consequence of it. This means that it will not only make you lean and fit but will also make you healthy.

SOME OF THE important health benefits of the OMAD routine

Weight Loss without a Calorie Restrictive Diet

Obesity has become a global issue. It is killing more people on a worldwide scale than most of the calamities combined. This has opened up a massive market for the weight loss industry, and it is flourishing rapidly. There are scores of popular diets and ways that promise weight loss. However, I have presented the facts in the earlier chapters that the stats tell a completely different story. Obesity is increasing at an alarming rate year after year. This doesn't mean that those diets don't work at all. They certainly do! However, most of the diets are unsustainable in the end.

If you have been a prolific junk eater for most of your life, then switching entirely to a leafy diet will not only be painful but soul-crushing too. People start feeling sad, depressed, and irritated. The day they return to their regular diet, they try to compensate for the loss of the taste by binge eating. The weight gain comes back faster than they had lost it. Studies show that most people who lost weight through diets regained more than they had lost. This problem cannot be ignored.

Another problem that plagues people on fad diets is the fact that most of the weight they lose is water weight. You limit the number of calories in the diet as well as some of the nutrients. This leads to water loss. It may appear that you have lost some weight, but in reality, it is misleading and a delusion. As soon as you get back to your normal routine, the water weight would come back.

The OMAD routine leads to substantial and sustainable weight loss that is easy to maintain. The primary reason for this success lies in the fact that it is a complete lifestyle change. The weight loss occurs because you rectify the things that cause obesity. Therefore, you can lose weight and maintain it with great ease and success. Another important factor is that the OMAD routine doesn't put a calorie restriction. You are free to eat whatever healthy things you like in a moderate manner. You can also have you cheat days when you can literally eat anything. The major shift that comes with OMAD routine is with the timing of your meal and fast. When you allow your body ample time to digest the food and metabolize the fat, only then does the real weight loss occur. This is the working principle behind the OMAD routine. You get one meal in a day. You can eat whatever you like. However, for the rest of the time, your body gets the time to burn the extra fat in your body as fuel. This makes weight relapse a difficult proposition as you have already lost it.

Helpful in Diabetes

Diabetes is without a doubt another major problem of this world. People mostly try to justify their diabetes as a genetic disorder. In most cases, it's untrue. Even if your parents have carried diabetes-causing genes, diabetes doesn't begin out of thin air. Your poor lifestyle and poor food choices help it emerge intensely and quickly. You can keep diabetes at bay even if it has been in your family lineage. However, this is only for those people who inherited diabetes from their parents. For most of the diabetic patients, this isn't the case. Diabetes is usually a lifestyle disorder for most. Uncontrolled sugar and fast food, frequent eating, insulin spikes, and a sedentary lifestyle can cause diabetes in anyone. It is easy to blame other things as a scapegoat for your actions. However, the solution can only come when you own the situation and take responsibility. You will need to take remedial steps because the next stop after diabetes is obesity.

Interestingly, even obesity can easily lead to diabetes. Both of these problems are tightly interconnected. If you have one, then you have a very high risk of the other.

The OMAD routine of intermittent fasting can help you both in diabetes and obesity. It can also help you in avoiding them altogether. The OMAD routine improves your insulin sensitivity and reduces insulin resistance. This brings your blood sugar levels in control. You can burn your fat more efficiently and lose weight fast. It addresses the root of the problem and gives great relief in diabetes. If you are on the verge of diabetes or you have pre-diabetes, then the OMAD routine can help you in preventing diabetes. If you already have diabetes, then it can help you in reversing the effects of diabetes.

Remember, obesity and diabetes are tightly linked together. Your obesity may only be the effect of your diabetes. You can get great help from the OMAD routine in that case. It stabilizes your blood glucose levels and makes your body burn the extra fat. If your blood glucose levels remain stable and you do not have diabetes, then your chances of becoming obese also reduced to a safe level.

Better Management of Blood Pressure

One big benefit of the OMAD routine is a reduction in the intake of processed food. It is a blessing in disguise. Although the OMAD routine gives you the flexibility to eat almost anything you want, you would want to keep a healthy diet as it will be your only meal of the day. This takes away most of the processed and fast food from your menu. These items are packed with artificial sweeteners and sodium in various forms. Sodium leads to a lot of water retention in your body. This leads to an abnormal increase in blood pressure.

Blood pressure may not look like a big problem for many, but it is a silent killer like other lifestyle disorders. It will affect your heart as well as your body. It acts like a slow poison and brings your body down. A nagging headache, irritation, anger, excitability, compromised heart, and kidney function are some of the problems caused by increased blood pressure. It will slow you down and make your life difficult.

The OMAD routine helps by eradicating the primary cause of high blood pressure from your diet, i.e. high sodium food.

With controlled blood pressure, your metabolic function remains proper. Your heart and kidneys work in order, and it becomes easier for you to maintain weight.

Lowers Oxidative Stress and Free Radical Damage

Oxidation and accumulation of free radicals in the blood is a steady process. When your body continuously burns carbohydrates, free radicals and oxidation increase in the body. This process, among other things, leads to aging. Early signs of aging are a direct result of high oxidative stress and free radical damage. Anti-aging creams and procedures may hide the signs of aging, but they can't hide the fact that your body is under stress.

The **OMAD** routine presents an easy solution to this problem. When you start the **OMAD** routine, your body cannot rely only on the carbohydrate fuel, as it is in short supply. It starts burning the fat fuel. The burning of fat releases very few free radicals as it is a comparatively cleaner fuel, consequently reducing the toxic waste accumulation in your body.

The **OMAD** routine also leads to the generation of antioxidants in considerable amounts. These antioxidants help in reducing oxidative stress. Antioxidants also greatly help in reducing free radical damage. This single advantage is reason enough to adopt an OMAD routine. People spend a fortune on looking young and beautiful. They want longevity and vitality. Reducing the oxidative stress and free radical damage can do all this for you, naturally.

If you feel you are looking more and more haggard with the passage of time and you want to look magnificent and charismatic, then adopt the **OMAD** routine for results.

Improvement of Cholesterol Levels

Cholesterol is advertised as the big villain in our body. Everyone wants to get rid of cholesterol, but little do they know that it performs some most critical functions. It is the building block of several hormones and the structure of your cells. If it weren't for cholesterol, even producing sex hormones wouldn't be possible for your body. Your brain is the hungriest organ for cholesterol. Your endocrine, adrenal, and sex glands also need cholesterol for producing the critical hormones like testosterone and progesterone. The digestive bile acids in your intestine are also made from cholesterol. Cholesterol also allows the production of vitamin D in your body.

There are mainly two types of cholesterol present in your body. The HDL or the good one and the LDL or the bad one. It is the imbalance in the levels of both of these cholesterols that causes problems. Heart problems become a significant concern if the LDL increases in your body. This LDL is deposited in your arteries easily and causes the blockage.

There is a popular misconception that you can lower the cholesterol levels by merely reducing the dietary intake of cholesterol. In principle, this sounds correct. However, while you reduce the levels of LDL, the HDL levels also go down automatically and therefore, no positive impact can be enjoyed.

Your body is producing cholesterol in ample quantity. It can also burn the LDL effectively while preserving the HDL levels for better heart function. You can make this happen with the help of intermittent fasting.

During intermittent fasting, our liver starts burning the fat fuel. It uses up free fatty acids to produce energy. The triacylglycerol synthesis goes low at this stage and in turn, leads to lower levels of VLDL. This whole process ultimately leads to reduced production of LDL. The levels of HDL usually remain the same in the body and hence the positive functions of cholesterol remain unaffected.

If you have high cholesterol levels, you can end up taking massive doses of cholesterol reducing pills like 'Statin.' However, the overall situation for you remains the same, and you get dependent on medicine. The LDL deposit in your arteries keeps drawing you near to an impending heart attack. The best way to avoid this problem is to follow intermittent fasting.

Intermittent fasting helps your liver in burning the fat fuel. It is a cleaner and better fuel. The production of LDL, VLDL, and triglycerides will also go down, and you won't have to face so many problems.

Improved Heart Health

The heart is one of the most important organs in our body. It pumps blood into your body and keeps you alive. However, it is a sensitive organ. Your lifestyle can have an adverse impact on your heart beside the negative effect of high levels of cholesterol and blood pressure.

The stress and panic of the current era are putting pressure on our hearts more than anything else. The heart starts aging fast, and the blood vessels get stiff. Intermittent fasting and exercise can immensely help such people. When you exercise during intermittent fasting, your body produces a lot of Nitric oxide. It helps in relaxing the blood vessels. The relaxed blood vessels widen and can carry more blood. This whole process is called vasodilation.

Chronic stress in the current age comes as a package deal. The more successful you are, the higher the pressure will be. Medicines will treat the symptoms but do nothing about the cause. Intermittent fasting helps you in releasing the stress. Intermittent fasting helps you not only by reducing the stress on your muscles but also calms your mind and spirit.

Better Brain Function

The brain is the most influential and vital organ in your body. You can't function without a brain even for a bit. If its function is impaired even slightly, your functionality drops drastically. The best thing about the brain is that it isn't static. There is furious activity going in it all the time. This leads to degeneration. Cells get overworked, old, and damaged. However, our brain also has the capability of regenerating cells. This process is called neuro-plasticity.

However, this ability to regenerate cells in the brain is dependent on a unique neurotrophic factor called brain-derived neurotrophic factor (BDNF). The production BDNF needs a stimulus. Intermittent fasting provides that stimulus to your brain. Several studies have demonstrated that the production of BDNF can go up by 50 to 400 percent during intermittent fasting. The increase of the growth varies from one region of the brain to the other.

Nevertheless, the impact of intermittent fasting on BDNF and eventually on neuroplasticity is clear. It leads to better memory, regeneration, adaptation and improved neural connections. Studies are going on to find out if it can also help in neurodegenerative disorders like Alzheimer's and Parkinson's diseases. Still, the positive impact on the brain is evident.

Powerful Immune System

People find it hard to believe, but the most of our immune system is in our gut. Frequent eating and unhealthy food can cause considerable damage to the immune system in our intestine and cause several problems. When we eat too frequently, we do not give our gut the time to recover. Unhealthy food also causes significant damage to the gut bacteria, and our immune system gets very weak. Frequent bouts of a cough, cold, allergies or infections are a result of the weak immune system.

The OMAD routine gives your gut the chance to recover from the onslaught of food you ate 20 hours ago. This is a reasonable period for its recovery. It also gives a boost to autophagy which is a system of self-repair and maintenance.

After a few days of following the OMAD routine, you'll find that your wounds have started recovering fast and you are less prone to seasonal allergies. This is the beginning of a fit, and healthy life as your body will be able to strengthen its protective mechanism.

Freedom from Lethargy and Grogginess

One of the most common problems of obese people is that they continuously feel lethargic and groggy. They feel tired even after waking up from sleep and keep hitting the snooze button. They are unsteady all the time and are unsure of their strength. The high glucose level in their blood is mainly responsible for this problem. Carbohydrate-rich diets keep pumping glucose into their bloodstream, and their body continues storing it as fat. Their metabolic rate decreases and they keep feeling the need to conserve more energy. The fat burning mechanism in their body goes to sleep, and so do they. This largely contributes towards their complacent lifestyle and attitude.

However, the OMAD routine can help in this area too. The OMAD routine helps in stabilizing the blood sugar levels and starts burning fat in the body. The clean energy released by fat burning gives a significant boost to energy levels. Their body starts burning the fat and their metabolic rate increases. This also helps in reducing the overall weight too.

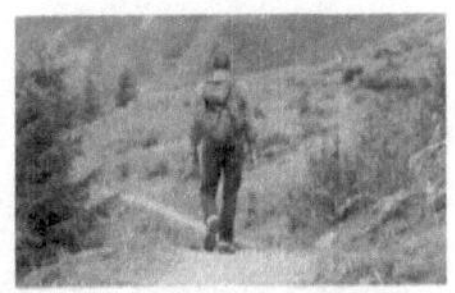

Conclusion

Thanks for making it through to the end of this book; let's hope it was informative and able to provide you with all of the tools you need to achieve your weight loss goals.

The OMAD routine of intermittent fasting is the best way to lose weight fast and in the right manner. It gives a major boost to your body and health. You lose not only a lot of water weight but also the tough belly fat.

The OMAD routine can make your life easy and make you feel more positive about yourself. It is a sustainable routine that is easy to follow. You can lead any lifestyle, and this routine would easily fit into it. You will lose weight safely and quickly, which is why it's so popular.

If you are tired of carrying the extra weight on your body and the belly fat makes you look bad, then adopt the OMAD routine. If health concerns bother you, then following the OMAD routine is best. This routine will help you achieve your target BMI and overall health biomarkers.

Your body is an amazing machine. It has the capability of curing most problems and keeping you healthy. Your irregular eating patterns and constant abuse of food damages the healing system. The OMAD routine helps in restoring the self-healing mechanism and activates autophagy. You can get a healthy body and anti-aging effects by following the OMAD routine.

This book has tried to explain the process of the OMAD routine and the good things it has in store for you. It will help you in your weight loss journey and guide you in the correct ways to achieve optimal health.

Finally, if you found this book useful in any way, a review on Amazon is always appreciated!